ONCE A MONTH

❧

"Dr. Dalton's book was the first in America to explain what PMS is and offer treatment hope to sufferers. She continues to bring out valuable new and updated information with each edition. ONCE A MONTH was the best book in the beginning and still is today. I highly recommend it to all women who suffer from PMS and their doctors."
    —Marla Ahlgrimm, R.Ph., Founder/President of Women's Health America Foundation and Co-founder of PMS Access

"This is the first thing I recommend to women with premenstrual syndrome. It reassures women who suffer, gives clear information, and suggests concrete solutions. It's invaluable for women and for everyone whose lives they touch."
    —Virginia Cassara, Executive Director, PMS Action, Inc.

"ONCE A MONTH is the single most important book I have ever read. It certainly saved my sanity and quite possibly my life. You can't know how grateful I am to you—and the gratitude is profoundly shared by my husband and our son."
    —M. T. I., Waynesburg, Pa.

"This book is written with the aim of spreading the news that the once-a-month miseries of countless women can be, and are being, successfully treated and relieved. It is also written to help men understand and appreciate the menstrual problems of women, and become partners in helping them through their difficult days. That you are reading this book brings hope that the aim will be achieved."
    —From the Book

ONCE A MONTH
Understanding and Treating PMS

— ❧ —

KATHARINA DALTON, M.D.
With Wendy Holton

Hunter House
PUBLISHERS

Hunter House Inc., Publishers
P.O. Box 2914
Alameda CA 94501-0914

Library of Congress Cataloging-in-Publication Data

Dalton, Katharina, 1916–
Once a Month: understanding and treating PMS
Katharina Dalton with Wendy Holton. — 6th rev. ed.
p. cm.
Includes bibliographical references and index.
ISBN 0-89793-255-2. — ISBN 0-89793-256-0
1. Premenstrual syndrome. 2. Menstruation disorders. I. Holton, Wendy. II. Title.
RG165.D34 1999
618.1'72—dc21 99-10080
CIP

Project credits

Cover Design: Peri Poloni
Project Editors: Kiran Rana,
Jennifer Rader
Managing Editor: Wendy Low
Proofreader: Lee Rappold
Publicity: Marisa Spatafore

Book Design: *Qalagraphia*
Copy Editor: Rosana Francescato
Acquisitions Coordinator:
Jeanne Brondino
Indexer: Kathy Talley-Jones
Marketing Intern: Monique Portegies

Customer Support: Christina Sverdrup, Joel Irons
Order fulfillment: A & A Quality Shipping Services
Publisher: Kiran S. Rana

9 8 7 6 5 4 3 2 1   Sixth Edition   99 00 01 02 03

Contents

List of Figures

About the Author

Katharina Dalton was born in England in 1916. Her early training was as a chiropodist at the London Foot Hospital, where she wrote *Essentials of Chiropody*, now a basic textbook. Widowed with one child during the war, she started medical training at the Royal Free Hospital, worked in the evenings, remarried, and had three more children. In 1948 she qualified as an M.D. and entered general practice, where, during the first two months, she identified and successfully treated six women suffering from premenstrually related asthma, epilepsy, and migraine. For fifty years she has continued researching premenstrual syndrome in her extensive practice. This interest resulted in 1953 in the first paper in British medical literature on premenstrual syndrome, written in collaboration with Dr. Raymond Greene. In 1954 her work with premenstrual syndrome patients at University College Hospital, London, led to her establishing there the world's first premenstrual syndrome clinic, which she closed in 1996. She continues her work in her Harley Street practice, while also continuing to study and lecture on premenstrual syndrome, postnatal depression, and related illnesses.

Dr. Dalton is now an acknowledged authority on the part played by menstrual dysfunctions in confused and criminal behavior, accidents, drug abuse, and morbidity. Her work on premenstrual syndrome and its treatment with progesterone therapy is applied in factories, schools, prisons, shops, and hospitals, and she has received widespread recognition for her research. She has been awarded the Charles Oliver Hawthorne BMA prize for outstanding research in general practice on three occasions, and she has also received the Upjohn Fellowship, the Charlotte Brown prize, and the Cullen prize from the Royal Free Hospital, and the British Migraine Association prize from the Royal College of General Practitioners, of which she was a founding member. In 1971 she became the first woman president of the General Practice section of the Royal Society of Medicine. In 1980 she was expert witness in two cases of murder in which premenstrual syndrome was first accepted as a factor causing diminished responsibility, thus making legal history in England. She was awarded the Fellowship of the Royal College of General Practitioners in 1982.

Her books and publications have been translated into sixteen languages and include *The Premenstrual Syndrome* (1964), *The Menstrual Cycle* (1969), *The Premenstrual Syndrome and Progesterone Therapy* (1977, 2d ed. 1984), *Depression After Childbirth* (1980, 3d ed. 1996), *Premenstrual Syndrome Illustrated* (1990), *Premenstrual Syndrome Goes to Court* (1990), and *PMS: The Essential Guide to Treatment Options* (1994). She has lectured extensively to both medical and lay audiences all over the world and has made numerous radio and TV appearances in Europe, the United States, Australia, and Singapore.

Her husband, the Reverend Tom Dalton, a Unitarian minister, died after forty-eight years of marriage. He was part of a team with his wife, working to help sufferers of premenstrual syndrome, ghostwriting her books, and helping the families of sufferers to understand the problems. Dr. Dalton's family are all involved in her work. She has two sons and two daughters: Michael is a general practitioner, Tony is responsible for her computing skills, Wendy is her co-author, and Maureen is a consultant gynecologist. One of her five grandchildren, Jennie, wrote chapter 12 of this book, and another, Sarah, is a medical student.

About the Co-author, Wendy Holton

In the days before computers were commonplace, the collation of information for statistics was child's play. While still at school, Wendy spent many a vacation or Sunday afternoon playing a kind of Happy Families game. It was a simple method of sorting into groups the point in a woman's menstrual cycle when incidents occurred, such as hospital admission, accidents, childhood visits to the doctor, and so on, to provide the statistics contained in the papers her mother, Katharina Dalton, had published on the effects of premenstrual syndrome.

On leaving school Wendy trained as a secretary and worked in that field in London; this talent proved useful in typing all her mother's publications over the years, until the widespread use of PCs in the late '80s. By that time she was office manager of Katharina Dalton's private practice, arranging research projects from the first seed of an idea to implementation and final publication, as well as having day-to-day contact with the patients. In the mid-90s she gained a diploma in integrative counseling, which she combined with her work with sufferers of premenstrual syndrome.

As a sufferer of PMS herself, she understands the frustration experienced by so many when the "monster takes over" a normally placid woman. She is a talented cake maker, but alas, in those few premenstrual days before she was able to control her PMS, the cakes burned and ended up in the trash can rather than the cake tin. Through diet, she has successfully managed to keep that monster at bay for over three decades.

When Katharina Dalton appeared for five minutes on a British television show in 1991, the producers were rightly concerned about the viewers who would call up asking for help with their own PMS. Wendy was persuaded to provide an information network for these anxious viewers, and she started PMS Help. Within twenty hours of Katharina Dalton's five-minute televised item, over 470 inquiries were received through the mail, this number mounting to over 4,000 within the first week. As the inquiries continued pouring in, there were 10,000 in that first month. PMS Help became a national registered charity, offering postal information and support to sufferers of premenstrual syndrome, and also their families, being conscious of the effects PMS has not only upon the sufferer but also on all those with whom she comes into contact. Wendy has been chairman of PMS Help since its formation in 1991.

Although she moved away from London to a more rural life with her husband in 1996, she continues with her work in helping sufferers of premenstrual syndrome. She hopes that all readers of this book will gain a greater understanding of exactly what PMS is and how it can easily be controlled.

Preface to First Edition

This book is dedicated to the thousands of women who have confided in me the most personal and intimate details of their lives and from whom I have learned so much.

I am deeply grateful for the help received from all my family. To Drs. Maureen and Michael Dalton who have been my most severe critics; to Mrs. Anita Dalton and Mrs. Wendy Holton who have patiently typed, corrected, and retyped the manuscript before it was ready for submission to the publishers; to my niece Mrs. Sherryl Machray for the artwork; to Mrs. Sharlynn Orr who has kindly adapted my work for America; and most of all to my long-suffering husband, Rev. Tom Dalton, for his invaluable ghostwriting of the entire book.

Finally, my acknowledgment to David Duff and Tandem Press for the excerpt from *Albert & Victoria,* and the *Journal of the Royal College of General Practitioners* for their permission to reproduce Figure 11.

Katharina Dalton
1978

Preface to the Sixth Edition

The need for yet another edition of this book reflects the numerous scientific advances of the last few years that have been related to the problems of PMS. The development of nuclear medicine by molecular scientists has unraveled the mysteries of progesterone receptors. This is only the beginning—there is much more to be discovered and understood. The new paths of information have sped up its dissemination, enabling scientists worldwide to communicate and participate in the advances. This really is a new edition, but the aim remains the same: to remove the unnecessary, recurring problems that have blighted so many lives, not only of women but also of men and children.

In the fifty years since I first treated PMS, and especially since the first edition appeared, there have been sociological changes involving women in the workplace, altered dietary habits, and media influences. This has required new chapters: "Ups and Downs of Progesterone Therapy," "Hijacked by the Psychologists," "Normal Gynecological Examination," "Education and PMS," and "PMS and Contraception." There are also new chapters devoted to successful treatment: "Approach to Treatment," "Counseling for PMS," "The

Three-Hourly Starch Diet," "Rules of Progesterone Treatment," and "Psychiatric Treatment."

It is a great pleasure to introduce my daughter Mrs. Wendy M. Holton as my co-author. She has plenty of experience in observing PMS from a layperson's view. My son Tony and daughter Dr. Maureen have helped with the mysteries and marvels of the computer and e-mail, while my other son, Dr. Michael, has been engrossed with fighting the problems caused by the proposed legislation limiting the dose of vitamin B-6. My granddaughter, Jennie Holton, has written chapter 12, "PMS in Adolescence." It has ended up very much a family affair.

We are grateful to have received permission to reproduce the following figures:

Oxford University Press for permission to use Figures 17, 43, and 45 from my book *Depression After Childbirth*, 3rd Edition.

Thorsons for permission to use Figures 18, 20, 44, 46, 47, and 48 from my book *PMS: The Essential Guide to Treatment Options*.

The Lancet for Figures 22, 23, 32, and 33.

British Medical Journal for Figures 24, 25, and 26.

British Journal of Psychiatry for Figure 49.

Arun Krishna for allowing me to use Figures 30 and 31 from his M.S. project, 1992–1993.

My thanks are also extended to Rosana Francescato and Jennifer Rader of Hunter House, for so ably converting the British manuscript to a readable American book. So far I've only chatted with them on the phone and by e-mail.

Katharina Dalton
January 1999

1

———————— ૱ ————————

Introduction

Once a month, with monotonous regularity, chaos is inflicted on American homes as premenstrual tension and other premenstrual problems recur time and time again. Wonderfully happy and often long-term marriages and partnerships break up under the strain, because one partner is an unpredictable, irrational, or violent woman suffering from premenstrual syndrome (PMS). This book explains the many varied presentations of PMS, how it can be recognized and correctly diagnosed, and most important, how it can be successfully treated. It has been described as the world's most common disease, but too often it is not recognized before it has caused untold misery. This book has been written to help not only the sufferers but also their partners, families, friends, co-workers, and neighbors to understand how PMS can be recognized, correctly diagnosed, and successfully treated.

It has also been written to help men, as well as women, to understand the cause of these capricious and temperamental changes in women. The image of women as uncertain, fickle, changeable, moody, and hard to please needs to be replaced with the recognition that all these features can be understood in terms of the ever-changing ebb and flow of a woman's menstrual hormones and the hormonal changes they cause within her body cells. It is estimated that over 5.5 million American women suffer from monthly problems that can and should be relieved.

For PMS to be properly appreciated it must be recognized in its full variety. Following a television documentary on PMS showing four situations—an alcoholic, a baby batterer (see *Dina*, pages 254–255), a husband beater, and a neurotic—the hospital mailbox was filled with letters suggesting the program had been an eye-opener to many viewers. The letters contained such comments as

> It was such a relief to know that so many other women experience the very real and deep feelings of anger, hatred, and depression that I feel before my period.

> I am just like that woman.

> I never told anyone because I thought they would never believe me.

BRITISH NATIONAL HEALTH SERVICE

In 1948, the British National Health Service (NHS) started giving free medical care from the cradle to the grave. I was a newly qualified M.D. working in a poor North London suburb, where previously doctors had been too expensive for the residents, so pharmacists performed as best they could without examining, or even seeing, the patient. In August 1948 I came across my first case of premenstrual asthma, which responded successfully to treatment with progesterone injections. Before the month had passed, I had found a further case of asthma, two of epilepsy, and two of migraines that all occurred just before menstruation. They also responded successfully to progesterone. Together with Dr. Raymond Greene (brother of author Graham Greene) I continued to find more cases of PMS, and in 1953 we published in the *British Medical Journal* the first paper in medical literature describing the many bodily premenstrual presentations, as well as tension, and gave it the name "premenstrual syndrome."

Under the NHS, general practitioners were allowed to prescribe any drugs needed, but no toiletry or food. This meant that I was able to give progesterone treatments to all my diagnosed PMS patients. Every year our prescribing costs were studied, and those practitioners whose costs were above average received a visit from the Man from the Ministry, who discussed costs and ways in which they could be reduced. Those doctors persistently overprescribing after being advised three times were entitled to be heard by a tribunal before being fined. So in 1958 I attended the first ever NHS Tribunal on Over Prescribing and was judged by a barrister, a professor of obstetrics from Liverpool, and a general practitioner from Birmingham. The Medical Defence Union defended me superbly. The problem arose from my prescribing progesterone for thirty-five PMS patients during one specified month. Their full medical records were available showing their menstrual charts, previous suicide attempts, mental hospital admissions, and normal gynecological examinations. Finally the tribunal agreed that "progesterone is reasonable and necessary treatment for premenstrual syndrome." They did add that mine was not an average practice as it had more females than males (surprised?), that if all doctors prescribed as I did the cost of progesterone would go down, but that if all doctors prescribed progesterone to all their patients with PMS immediately the cost to the nation would equal the annual defense budget. The announcement was low-key, the media of the day did not cover it, and I continued treatment of an ever-increasing caseload of PMS patients.

Surveys in North London showed that the attempted suicide rate increased sevenfold for women who were in the second half of their menstrual cycle, and shoplifting was thirty times more common in women who were in the second half of the cycle. In 1977 it was found that of the 132 women attending the Premenstrual Syndrome Clinic at University College Hospital,

London, 37 percent had a previous psychiatric hospital admission, 34 percent had attempted suicide or homicide, 9 percent had alcoholic bouts, 6 percent were referred because of actual child abuse, a further 4 percent sought treatment because they feared that their injuries to their children would become public knowledge, 6 percent had a history of criminal behavior, such as smashing windows and assaulting police, 7 percent had premenstrual epilepsy, and 5 percent had premenstrual asthma. These are not trivialities but matters of vital concern to the patient, her family, society, and even the nation. But it was not until a PMS arsonist was freed on probation in 1979 and two PMS murderers were freed on probation that Americans started to take the many problems of PMS seriously.

FIFTY YEARS OF CHANGES

In the fifty years since PMS was first recognized, there have been unforeseen sociological changes, as well as scientific advances and new drugs, which have influenced the treatment of PMS.

In the forties, antidepressants had not been developed, so barbiturates were used in excess. There were no sleeping tablets, but liquid chloral hydrate was used, which gave mental hospitals their peculiar smell that permeated everywhere. There were no oral diuretic tablets, only Mersalyl injections used sparingly for cardiac edema, never for bloatedness. Progesterone could be administered only by deep intramuscular injections in the buttock; the suppository for vaginal or rectal use had not been developed. The contraceptive pill had not been developed.

The thalidomide disaster awakened the medical profession to the harm of drugs given during pregnancy. The artificial progestogens used in contraceptive pills were found to cause masculinization of the female fetus. The differences between natural progesterone and artificial progestogens were not generally recognized, so the use of progesterone during pregnancy was stopped (progesterone had been used to prevent threatened and habitual miscarriages, as well as preeclampsia). It was

Doctors Steptoe and Roberts who realized that progesterone was essential to the success of in vitro fertilization, and then progesterone once again achieved respectability and could be used during pregnancy.

Progesterone levels used to be measured from their breakdown product, pregnenalone, in a day's collection of urine. This was recognized as a fairly inaccurate test, because an unknown amount of progesterone was also excreted in the feces. The development of the accurate hormone measurements from blood samples by radioimmunoassays was a leap forward in our medical knowledge, but it did bring to light the fact that PMS subjects do not always have a low progesterone level in the premenstruum, the days immediately prior to menstruation. This was enough for many to stop progesterone therapy, as it could no longer be shown to be needed. It allowed PMS to be hijacked by the psychologists (see chapter 9). Meanwhile, other scientists, the molecular biologists, were benefiting from electron microscopes and studying the characteristics of progesterone receptors. In particular, they noted that progesterone receptors could not transport molecules of progesterone to the nucleus of cells in the presence of adrenaline. The usual time for an adrenaline release to occur is when the blood sugar level drops, so now it is realized that to prevent PMS one must avoid a drop in blood sugar; hence the development of the Three-Hourly Starch Diet (see chapter 24).

Scientists have also shown that a small amount of progesterone is present in both sexes from early fetal life until death. It is present in the inner lining cells of our blood vessels, where it ensures smoothness; in our bones, to prevent osteoporosis; in the myelin layer around our nerves; in our brain cells, where it is involved in the dopamine pathway controlling emotions; and in our lungs, skin, and hair follicles.

The sociological changes that have affected PMS over the last half century include the move from the kitchen to the workplace for most women, contraception that allows women to plan and have their children later, increased marital stress and divorce, recognition of child abuse, greater mobility, and changes in nuclear families.

Women trying to fulfill maternal responsibilities plus work commitments often space their meals too far apart, which results in an inevitable increase in PMS (see chapter 24).

The next chapter will discuss exactly what PMS is, and later chapters will discuss how to recognize it.

2

*

What Is PMS?

There has been such a lack of a definition of PMS that in my 1984 book *The Premenstrual Syndrome and Progesterone Therapy* I insisted that PMS be defined at the beginning of every chapter. The editor did not like this unusual approach initially but finally allowed it. The definition I used was this one: PMS is the recurrence of symptoms before menstruation with complete absence of symptoms after menstruation.

PREMENSTRUAL SYNDROME
is
RECURRENCE of symptoms BEFORE menstruation
with COMPLETE ABSENCE of symptoms
AFTER menstruation.

The definition includes several important facts. The recurrence should be noted for a minimum of two cycles and continually observed during treatment. The symptoms before menstruation should not be present for more than fourteen days before menstruation, which is the number of days from ovulation until menstruation. When Sadie produced a menstrual chart showing symptoms lasting eighteen days before menstruation she explained, "But I have a long cycle of thirty-six days." She thought that ovulation always occurred mid-cycle—and indeed it does for those whose cycles average twenty-eight days, but not for those with long cycles. The time from ovulation to menstruation averages fourteen days; it may well be shorter, but very rarely is it longer. The "complete absence" of symptoms after menstruation should be at least seven days, although it may well last longer

It is also important to remember that the definition of PMS requires not only the presence of symptoms related to menstruation but also the complete absence of these symptoms at other times of the menstrual cycle. This complete absence should be present for at least seven days, although it may well last longer. It is the absence of symptoms and the change of mood after menstruation back to a happier, energetic feeling of normalcy that clinches the diagnosis. This letter from a patient illustrates the point:

> I suffered from the usual premenstrual symptoms for five years, and my tension, irritability, and depression were blamed on nerves. I must say I could never understand this, as it was only at certain times of the month that I seemed to be so nervous, tense, depressed, and lacking in confidence. I found that about ten to twelve days before my period I felt as if something was draining out of me, and as if something chemical was happening. So often I tried to pull myself together at this time and it just never worked. I get so irritable and nervous a week before menstruation that I just want to shut myself up in the house; I feel as if I can't go out to work, and I avoid any sort of social engagement at this time of the month. At other times I'm okay.

In the definition of PMS, no mention is made of the type of symptoms. This is because the symptoms vary; I described some 150 different symptoms in my 1964 book *The*

Premenstrual Syndrome, the first book ever published on the subject. Some of these are discussed in the next two chapters.

WARNING SENSATIONS

Before normal bodily functions are about to take place, Nature gives us valuable warning sensations. There are sensations that tell us when our bladder is full or our bowels need opening. We get a peculiar nasal tickling before sneezing, we feel thirsty when dehydrated, and we have a rumbling tummy when hungry. In the same way there are valuable and personal warning sensations before the start of menstruation. The sensations before menstruation should not be considered symptoms, although this thinking does account for the findings of some PMS surveys, which give an incidence of PMS exceeding 90 percent of those surveyed.

I learned the importance of warning sensations early in my career when I treated Diana, then thirty-six years old. A blind woman, she was an alert and intelligent counselor and had kept a Braille menstrual chart, showing recurrence of headaches, bloatedness, and exhaustion limited to the premenstruum, which confirmed the diagnosis of PMS. She was treated with progesterone injections. At her next visit she brought her chart showing the days of menstruation and a complete absence of symptoms, but she was not a happy lady. She was furious, and she shouted in a high-pitched voice:

> There I was, walking out of a council meeting in my new gray suit with a plate-sized stain of red blood on my seat. No thanks—I would rather have a warning.

She was experiencing a complete absence of any warning sensation heralding the approach of menstruation. This is something that passes unnoticed in volunteers participating in double-blind placebo-controlled trials, because they are so busy keeping detailed reports of their symptoms that they are fully aware of the expected date of menstruation.

SEVERITY

The definition of PMS does not deal with the severity of symptoms, which may vary from mild, and welcome, warning sensations to severe suicidal depression. Treatment for PMS usually is limited to those with symptoms severe enough to interfere with their normal working or social life. There is a remarkable individual variation in PMS: no two patients are alike, and each patient requires individual attention.

The duration of PMS varies enormously. It may last a full fourteen days, with deep depression at ovulation lasting until a sudden ending when menstrual bleeding starts, while those prone to epileptic seizures caused by PMS may find that the devastating attack is measured in minutes or hours, not days. But both are deserving of treatment. Symptoms of migraine, psychosis, hallucinations, and alcoholic bouts tend to last only a day or two and come immediately before menstruation. Symptoms are always at their worst immediately before menstruation, and one is suspicious of those whose charts show a day or two of normalcy immediately before menstruation.

WE ARE ALL DIFFERENT

Women are different in so many ways: personal and facial characteristics, personality, parentage, family size and position, environment, education, previous illnesses, reactions to food and to drugs. So it is no surprise to find that women are also different in their menstrual patterns and their reactions to menstrual symptoms.

Men are also different. The range of responses shown by men to women with PMS and menstrual problems runs the gamut from genuine sympathy and understanding to annoyance, amazement, anger, aggression, disbelief, ridicule, and withdrawal. There is even the unthinking partner who says, "You've had it long enough, you ought to know how to deal with it" or "It can't be PMS, you had that last month."

NORMAL VARIATIONS OF MENSTRUATION

Just as there are numerous variations in our hair, not only in the color but also in the curliness, thickness, oiliness, and length, so each woman's menstrual cycle is unique and individual in the type and duration of flow and in the cycle length. The menstrual flow, which is the disintegrated lining of the womb, may appear as a pink watery discharge or as thick red blood. It may be reddish-brown or black, and it may contain shreds or small blood clots. All these variations are normal and healthy.

The variation in the length of the menstrual cycle is also important in determining the timing of medication for menstrual problems. Some treatments for PMS suggest starting on Day 12 and continuing until Day 26, but this is of little value to the woman with a thirty-six-day cycle, who then receives no medication during the vital last ten days of her cycle. Clearly, there can be no standard dose or timing of treatment that will be appropriate to every woman suffering from PMS. Each woman requires a personal regimen of treatment for success.

There are also variations in the amount of menstrual flow on different days of menstruation. Some women have the heaviest flow on the first, second, and third day and then stop abruptly. Others have moderate flow for a day or two and then the heaviest on the third or fourth day. Yet other women have a scanty flow for a day or two, with the flow gradually increasing in amount. It is important for the doctor to know the day of heaviest flow, because in PMS the spontaneous relief of symptoms will not occur until the full menstrual flow occurs.

It is important to appreciate that PMS can occur in cycles in which ovulation does not occur (anovular cycles), as well as in normal ovulatory cycles. Also, PMS can recur after recovery from the trauma of hysterectomy, with or without removal of both ovaries (see chapter 20).

MENSTRUAL MAGNIFICATION

Many women have mild symptoms throughout the cycle, which increase in severity in the premenstruum. This is known as *menstrual magnification* or *menstrual distress*. The symptoms after menstruation may represent a mere 5 percent of the symptoms during the premenstruum, or they may represent 90 percent of premenstrual symptoms. As there is no absence of symptoms after menstruation, the diagnosis cannot be PMS. Nevertheless, if the premenstrual symptoms are severe, menstrual distress is worth treating as PMS, but such patients should not be included in clinical trials for PMS.

3

⁂

The Diagnosis of PMS

Without a doubt, there is much confusion about PMS. Medical professionals are confounded by it, whether they are gynecologists, psychiatrists, or endocrinologists. Even family physicians, who see the condition first and are in an ideal situation for treating it, are perplexed. Few specialists know anything about it, even though PMS invades every specialty. Add to this the abysmal lack of knowledge about and experience with PMS revealed in the writings of an increasing number of lay authors, together with the appalling ignorance and utter befuddlement of the media's presentation on the subject, and it is only too easy to understand how the bewilderment continues to grow. I hope this chapter will clear away these mists of confusion.

First, it is essential to establish a definition of the disease in question in order to achieve a proper diagnosis. As mentioned in the previous chapter, the precise definition means that three requirements must be fulfilled for a correct diagnosis:

1. Symptoms must have been present every month for at least the previous two menstrual cycles.

2. Symptoms must be present premenstrually and cannot start before ovulation. (This means fourteen days or less before

menstruation; so in long cycles of thirty-six days, it will not start before day twenty-two.)

3. There must be a complete absence of symptoms after menstruation for a minimum of seven days.

The successful treatment of any disease depends on the accuracy of the diagnosis. To achieve that accuracy, a doctor must take three things into consideration: symptoms, signs, and investigations. That means the doctor listens to the patient's account of the complaint, takes note of any signs of disease that may be revealed by examination, and studies the results of blood tests, X rays, and other tests. The doctor accepts the patient's account of her symptoms (be they a sore throat or a pain in some other part of the body), and after examining for signs and considering the results of tests, makes the diagnosis and treats her accordingly. But all too often, when women come to their doctor claiming they have PMS, the doctor accepts their claim at face value without appreciating the need to check the diagnosis further before giving treatment.

TIME RELATIONSHIP OF SYMPTOMS TO MENSTRUATION

The doctor must verify the diagnosis of PMS, because there are no special symptoms indicative of the disease. The disease affects only women of childbearing age, but all its symptoms can also be experienced by men, children, and postmenopausal women. There are no specific signs discovered on examination and no definitive tests for it. How then to make an accurate diagnosis of a disease that has no special symptoms, no specific signs, and no distinctive tests? The one clear diagnostic clue is the time relationship of symptoms to menstruation. It is therefore necessary to use a method of diagnosis that enables this critical time relationship to be clearly established.

Psychiatrists frequently use questionnaires as part of their diagnostic procedures, asking the patient numerous questions and analyzing the replies. It allows numerical scores to be obtained for an individual's level of depression, anxiety, neuroticism, or marital stability. This score can then be used to compare the results of different treatments. This is a useful method for diagnosing psychological diseases, but not for PMS.

MENSTRUAL DISTRESS QUESTIONNAIRES

In 1968 Rudolph Moos designed a questionnaire that is very effective in demonstrating the amount of distress caused by menstruation, although it cannot differentiate PMS from menstrual pain or distress. In the Moos Menstrual Distress Questionnaire a woman is asked to answer forty-seven different questions each night on a six-point scale. These include questions such as "Today did you have any excitement? . . . loneliness?" It is a method that relies on the honesty, reliability, and determination of the candidate. While it may be easy to carefully consider your reply and complete the questionnaire for one—or even seven—consecutive days, one doubts the accuracy of the responses when, as in the tests conducted by Dr. Sampson in 1978 and 1988, women were asked to complete a questionnaire every single day for six months. Moreover, there is always a need for caution in interpreting the results of questionnaires when they are used for purposes other than those for which they were designed.

Incidentally, whenever I am conducting a clinical trial I insist on my helpers also completing a chart daily, as only then do they realize how easy it is to forget the task or fill it out inaccurately without really thinking about each question. Men can also fill out the questionnaires or charts, for they also have days when they feel lazy, irritable, or fed up. Unfortunately, the Moos Questionnaire concentrates on common psychiatric symptoms and does not cover all the possible 150 symptoms that may occur in PMS. Some useful questions that are missing include "Did you have a long interval between meals today?" "Did you have too much alcohol today?" "How many puffs of your inhaler did you need today to control your asthma?" "Could you wear your contact lenses today?" Furthermore, the questionnaires cannot be answered by those few severely ill patients who are temporarily confused, deluded, or hallucinating during the premenstruum but are free of symptoms during the postmenstruum.

It must not be forgotten that the information obtained from such questionnaires needs to be prospective, i.e., obtained daily, rather than retrospective, i.e., obtained by such questions as "During the days before menstruation do you suffer from . . . ?" Today, women have been educated by the media to know that tension, headaches, bloating, backache, and irritability tend to occur premenstrually. If they suffer from these symptoms at all, when thinking back to when the symptoms might have occurred, they may automatically assume that they occurred premenstrually.

Ramcharan and his colleagues in 1993 reported a study in which an interviewer recorded a questionnaire of symptoms on one specific day of the cycle. There were 1,677 women who refused to participate, but we cannot know how many of these suffered from severe PMS. Can one really expect a woman to agree to be interviewed after she has fought with her husband, battered the children, thrown items across the room, or crashed the car, or when she is confused and exhausted, breathless from asthma, vomiting from a migraine, recovering from an epileptic seizure, or aphonic from laryngitis? If the interview is postponed for one week the woman is then in her asymptomatic week, and again PMS will be missed. It must be recognized that PMS cannot be diagnosed by means of a one-day-only interview.

THE MENSTRUAL CHART

If the help of the patient is needed in making the diagnosis, it is important to keep the diagnostic aids simple to eliminate the possibility of inaccuracy and guesswork. The menstrual chart shown in Figure 1 is widely used by doctors and is easy enough for anyone to copy.

The purpose of the chart is to provide the precise information necessary to make an accurate diagnosis of PMS. This is done by recording the actual dates of menstruation and the days when symptoms or complaints are present. The woman is asked to choose only her three most important symptoms—those complaints she would most like to lose. These symptoms are then given symbols, such as H for headache, X for quarrels, T for tension. A small h, x, or t can be used for mild symptoms, and capital letters for symptoms that are really severe. There shouldn't be a need to use more than one letter for any one symptom. It does not matter what letters are used; for example, the letter M may be used to represent menstruation, but some use P for period. The chart is completed each night with a record of whether the symptom was present or absent, and whether it was severe during that day. Some women like to insert a dot on those days when they feel well. This ensures that they complete the record. The chart should be completed daily regardless of the phase of the menstrual cycle or the apparent cause of the symptom. Doctors interpreting the chart need to be aware that external circumstances may cause the same symptoms as PMS. For instance, a few hours spent watching your child having his lacerated leg sutured in an emergency room can cause you to feel tense, irritable, or depressed, regardless of the phase of your cycle. You may have every reason to feel exhausted or have a headache after your flight is delayed all night when you are returning from a vacation.

From a menstrual chart it immediately becomes obvious whether symptoms are clustered around menstruation, as in Figure 2, or occur haphazardly throughout the month, as in Figure 3. It is easy to see the duration of menstruation or of symptoms, and whether the menstrual cycle is short, when the M's will be going up the chart, or long, when the M's will be starting down the chart. It is also not necessary for the woman to be at a time of life when she is menstruating to obtain information about the cyclical character of her symptoms. Cyclical symptoms can occur before menstruation has begun, at times

Name _____ Year _____

	Jan.	Feb.	Mar.	Apr.	May	Jun.	Jul.	Aug.	Sep.	Oct.	Nov.	Dec.
1												
2												
3												
4												
5												
6												
7												
8												
9												
10												
11												
12												
13												
14												
15												
16												
17												
18												
19												
20												
21												
22												
23												
24												
25												
26												
27												
28												
29												
30												
31												

Figure 1   Simple menstrual chart

of occasional missed menstruation, at menopause, or even after removal of the womb or ovaries.

One mother, a sales executive who was herself receiving treatment for PMS, was disturbed to find that her thirteen-year-old daughter had occasional "off" days when she was rude and lazy, which was quite out of character for her. Then the mother received reports from school indicating that the girl had occasional rebellious days during which she found it hard to accept discipline. The mother carefully recorded the dates of these problems (shown on the chart in Figure 4), which occurred at intervals of thirty-two to thirty-six days. When the daughter later started to menstruate, the timing of her menstrual cycle

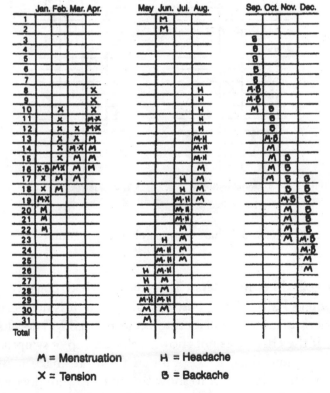

M = Menstruation   H = Headache
X = Tension   B = Backache

Figure 2   Menstrual charts diagnostic of premenstrual syndrome

	Jan.	Feb.	Mar.	Apr.	May	Jun.	Jul.	Aug.
1	X		X	M				H
2			X	M				
3			X	M	H	H		
4								
5				X				H
6				X	H		H	
7			M		H			
8	X	M·X				H		
9	X	M				H		
10		X	M			H		
11								H
12		M			M	H		
13		M	X	X	M			
14		M			M·H	H		
15		X			M		M	
16	X				M		M	
17	M				M		M	M
18	M				M	M	M	M
19	M	X			M	M	M	M
20		X		X		M	M	M
21			X			M	M	M
22			X		H	M		M
23	X				H	M		
24	X					M·H		
25	X							
26		X						
27				X				
28			X	M	H			H
29				M		H		
30	X			M			H	
31					H			
Total								

M = Menstruation   X = Quarrels
H = Headaches

Figure 3   Menstrual chart with unrelated symptoms

averaged thirty-five days. This mother had diagnosed her daughter's PMS before menstruation started. It is not necessary for menstruation or ovulation to occur before PMS develops.

If the chart does not show a relationship of symptoms to menstruation, there is no point in trying to make it fit the PMS pattern. It is wiser to show the chart to your doctor, as it may contain valuable clues that will indicate the true problem. It is not unknown for some women to copy a chart straight

	Jan.	Feb.	Mar.	Apr.	May	Jun.
1					X	
2						X
3						X
4						
5						X
6						
7						
8						
9						
10						
11						
12						
13						
14						
15						
16	X					
17	X	X				
18	X	X				
19						
20		X				
21	X	X				
22						
23		X				
24			X			
25			X			
26				X		
27			X	X		
28				X		
29			X	X		
30			X			
31					X	
Total						

Figure 4   Chart of adolescent girl with cyclical symptoms before the start of menstruation

from a book and then ask for help; unfortunately, in these circumstances there is little the doctor can do to help.

Occasionally, the diagnosis may be made by others whose
observations reveal the cyclical character of the symptoms.
For instance, a legal executive noted the days when her secretary's typing deteriorated and she became aggressive. When
these revealed a pattern of recurrence every thirty to thirty-six
days, the boss advised her secretary to seek medical help. The
value of similar information received from police, prison officers, and medical records is discussed in chapter 19.

HORMONE BLOOD TESTS

Tests to determine the blood level of progesterone are of little value in the diagnosis of PMS, for it is now known that the problem lies with the progesterone receptors rather than the level of progesterone in the blood, and there are as yet no routine investigations to determine the functioning of the progesterone receptors (see page 79). The secretion of progesterone from the corpus luteum of the ovary is intermittent and changes with marked variations within thirty minutes, so single blood samples taken on one day are of no help. It has recently been shown that the level of progesterone drops after big meals. Also, low levels of progesterone are found in women who are not ovulating, although they do not necessarily suffer from PMS.

However, a blood test to estimate the binding capacity of the sex hormone binding globulin (SHBG) has proved of some value in diagnosing premenstrual syndrome. My daughter, Dr. Maureen Dalton, showed in 1981 that fifty women suffering from severe, well-diagnosed PMS all had SHBG-binding levels below normal, compared with fifty healthy women, who were adamant that they did not suffer any premenstrual symptoms (see Figure 5). Furthermore, her tests showed that SHBG levels rise when progesterone is administered, and the greater the dose of progesterone the higher the SHBG level (see Figure 6). Later work showed that if progestogens were administered, the SHBG levels were lowered. It is now thought that SHBG is a reflection of hyperinsulinaemia. There are limitations on this test's usefulness, however, for the woman whose blood is to be tested must be free from all medication (which includes analgesics, oral contraceptives, laxatives, and vitamin preparations), must not be unduly obese or excessively hairy, and should not suffer from liver or thyroid disease. Furthermore, the blood must be centrifuged and stored frozen until analyzed by an elaborate method that is available only at a few specialized testing centers.

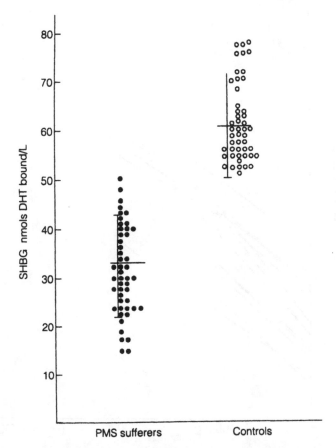

Figure 5 SHBG-binding capacity in fifty patients with severe premenstrual syndrome compared with fifty symptom-free controls

DIAGNOSTIC POINTERS OF PMS

Before a diagnosis of PMS can be made, women must complete the menstrual chart for two or three months. When selecting women for clinical trials on PMS, two-month's daily recording is the minimum, but sometimes a rough diagnosis is needed earlier. This can be done by considering characteristics that are common to most women with PMS and that differentiate

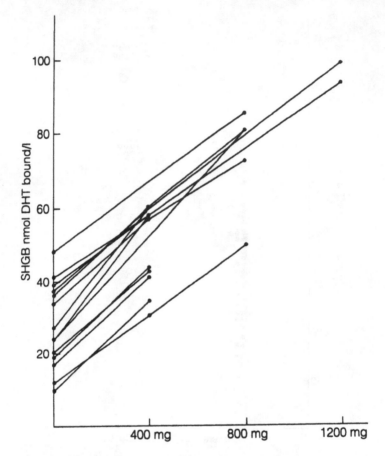

Figure 6   Effect of progesterone on SHBG levels

them from those who do not suffer from PMS. These characteristics are usually referred to as *diagnostic pointers*. The rest of
this chapter will deal with these characteristics and their usefulness as diagnostic pointers.

Medical students are taught that the onset of PMS is
linked with P-P-P-A: puberty, pregnancy, the Pill, and amenorrhea, or absence of menstruation, such as occurs during
anorexia nervosa, or after serious illnesses or accidents. In the
young adolescent, PMS may result in an unexpected change of
personality. One mother wrote,

For three weeks of the month our daughter is charming, capable, and intelligent; then for the few days before her period she is sharp-tongued, impossible to live with, and seems to be boiling with rage.

Spasmodic dysmenorrhea, or severe period pain, occurs only in ovulatory cycles and is unusual in PMS sufferers (see chapter 13). On the other hand, because their early periods are practically painless and uneventful, many young women with PMS initially fail to connect the symptoms in other parts of their body with menstruation.

Menstruation may stop unexpectedly when dieting, during a serious illness or accident, or when under great stress. When menstruation restarts, PMS frequently begins, or increases in severity.

During pregnancy menstruation does not occur, and the blood level of progesterone rises to thirty to fifty times the peak level reached during the premenstruum. At this time most women with PMS lose their symptoms. But even in symptom-free women, PMS may develop unexpectedly when menstruation returns after a pregnancy. If the pregnancy has been complicated by high blood pressure, swelling of the ankles, or an abnormally large gain in weight (signs of preeclampsia), or if it has been followed by postpartum or postnatal depression, then the chances are high—ten to one—that unpleasant premenstrual symptoms will follow in its wake. What is worse, the symptoms are likely to increase in severity after each pregnancy, even if later pregnancies are normal.

PMS may start when the woman is on the Pill, or during the week when she is off it, but complaints are likely to be more marked and the bright and dull days more accentuated when the woman stops taking the Pill and resumes her normal menstrual cycle. This cycle may well last three or five weeks, and not the precise twenty-eight days ordained by the makers of the Pill.

Marriage or the beginning of a relationship is often mentioned as a time when PMS starts, but it may be that the partner notices mood swings and other symptoms and relates them to menstruation, while the woman had not noticed the connection earlier. Again, taking the Pill may have coincided with the beginning of a relationship.

It is often an outside observer who first notices the mood swings, usually the partner or mother but occasionally an employer, social worker, friend, or child. Following a television broadcast on PMS, a husband wrote,

> I was so startled to recognize in all these cases the symptoms from which my wife has been suffering for the past eight years. The connection with the menstrual cycle may seem less direct but nevertheless her symptoms are heightened in the premenstrual period and free thereafter. Briefly, they include acute anxiety and depression (in any order, as it seems impossible to distinguish cause and effect) manifested by physical symptoms of pressure on the head (variously described as an iron band around the head or a heavy weight at the back of the head) and dizziness; and by psychological symptoms such as agoraphobia, panic, guilt, obsessions, and depression, sometimes to the extent of feeling suicidal.

It was first recognized by Radwanska, Hammond, and Berger of the University of Illinois, and later confirmed worldwide, that after women were sterilized by the simple operation to block their fallopian tubes, they subsequently produced less progesterone from their ovaries and their PMS increased in severity.

During adult life, PMS sufferers tend to have large weight swings exceeding twenty-eight pounds, although swings of fifty or more pounds are not unusual. The lowest weight since leaving school is subtracted from the highest nonpregnant weight to measure the adult weight swing. It is irrelevant whether the individual is obese or slim at the time the diagnosis is made.

PMS sufferers have difficulty in going long intervals without food, especially in the premenstruum. When they do, they may get faint, excessively tired, panicky, or irritable. They also tend to suffer from uncontrollable premenstrual food cravings and binges, especially when they have deliberately not eaten for a long time or when they have been dieting. This is not a personality failure but the result of the hormonal factor. It also occurs in baboons in the jungle, who climb the trees and in isolation gorge on unlimited amounts of honey during their premenstruum. And it was noticed that when rhesus monkeys at the Primate Center in Wisconsin were given precise numbers of pellets of food, their daily intake increased during the premenstruum.

Tolerance to alcohol also varies during the cycle in PMS sufferers. Although most days they can usually enjoy their favorite drink with no ill effects, during the premenstruum even a small amount causes intoxication.

Self-mutilation is another, more severe, less-common characteristic of the premenstruum. In severe cases of PMS, women have been known to slash their wrists, neck, abdomen, or face, burn themselves with cigarettes, or shave their hair and eyebrows.

Diagnostic Pointers of PMS

- Onset of PMS at a time of hormonal upset, e.g., at puberty, after pregnancy, after stopping the Pill, after a spell of amenorrhea, such as anorexia, or after a serious illness or accident.
- Pregnancy complicated by preeclampsia or postnatal depression.
- Large weight swings in adult life.
- Inability to tolerate long intervals without food.
- Inability to tolerate alcohol premenstrually.

- Increased libido premenstrually.
- Self-mutilation, such as slashing of the skin.

〜

If a woman gives many positive answers to the diagnostic pointers just listed, there is every likelihood that in two months she will return with a positive chart. There are occasions when it may be worth giving a patient a therapeutic trial with progesterone without waiting for a definitive diagnosis, but both the doctor and the patient should be aware that a positive diagnosis has not been made and the patient should not be included in a clinical trial. The evidence obtained from the diagnostic pointers may be accepted as evidence by the English courts for the diagnosis of PMS

An analysis was made of the final diagnosis in over two hundred women who attended a premenstrual clinic. Its conclusions were that while the menstrual chart is the only reliable diagnostic tool for PMS, the SHBG estimation was more specific, more sensitive, and had a greater predictive value than the checklist score of diagnostic pointers.

4

※

Symptoms of PMS

As I have mentioned, when discussing the definition of PMS we refer only to the timing of symptoms, without mentioning specific symptoms. This is because 150 different PMS symptoms have already been recorded, and no doubt there will be many more in the future. The symptoms cover the well-recognized tension and mood swings as well as more unusual symptoms, such as hair pulling and metatarsalgia. Because there are no specific symptoms of PMS, and all the symptoms can also occur in men, children, and postmenopausal women, it is the timing that clinches the diagnosis.

Already the symptoms seem to cover the majority of medical specialties. Apart from psychologists and gynecologists, also involved are urologists, ophthalmologists, physicians, surgeons, anesthetists, and cardiologists. When in general practice I soon appreciated that even geriatricians needed to be familiar with PMS. Many able caregivers have dutifully carried on the task of nursing an increasingly disabled, and probably incontinent, relative or friend, until one day they snap. Although a few days earlier they stated they were managing fine and needed no more help, suddenly they can manage no more. Everything is too much, and something must be done. The premenstruum is the time they snap, and often, help at that moment can solve the problem. By the next week they will have the energy and urge to carry on their wonderful work.

Characteristically, PMS patients have more than one system related to their symptoms, which is not surprising if it is agreed that PMS is a hormone-related disease, and progesterone receptors are present in most of the body's cells. So one patient may complain of depression, backache, and breast tenderness, and another of irritability, headache, and sweet cravings. They both have three symptoms involving different systems of the body.

The public tends to associate PMS with psychological symptoms, but in fact only one-third of the 150 symptoms are psychological. It is the psychological symptoms that are of greatest interest to the media, who enjoy reporting suicide attempts, admissions to drug clinics, and alcoholic binges of the famous but are not interested if someone misses a day's work because of a migraine attack.

There has been a marked change in the recognized PMS symptoms since its first description by Greene and Dalton in the *British Medical Journal* in 1953 compared with the symptoms reported to the FDA in 1982 when they were evaluating progesterone. While headaches topped the list in 1953, the later study showed an increase in depression, irritability, lethargy, and bloatedness. The later figures show the influence health education had on the reporting of breast tenderness (mastisis).

Comparison of Premenstrual Symptoms Reported in 1953 and 1982

Symptom	Greene and Dalton %	FDA %
Headache	69	33
Irritability	30	56
Depression	6	21
Lethargy	6	35
Vertigo	13	3
Skin and Mucosal Problems	13	3

Edema/Bloatedness	6	31
Rhinitis	7	1
Asthma	5	1
Epilepsy	5	3
Mastisis	2	21

TENSION

Tension may be described in many ways, but the tension that occurs in PMS has three parts to it: depression, tiredness, and irritability. These three aspects are always present in premenstrual tension, although one of them may be more obvious than the others, if only temporarily. Dr. Billig, in 1952, described the depression as feeling that "the world looks like a sour apple," the tiredness as "a fall in energy," and the irritability as "feeling crabby"—and there are plenty of women who know exactly what he meant.

```
PREMENSTRUAL TENSION
Is
DEPRESSION
and
TIREDNESS
and
IRRITABILITY
```

These three symptoms may be interwoven, with each one creating equal stress, as Dorothy's letter shows:

Premenstrual tension has been present throughout my reproductive life. I have seen my doctor many times but he has really been unable to help. Perhaps predictably, the condition had grown steadily worse in the years just before my marriage breakup, and has been much, much worse since. The strain is very great and practically unbearable during the premenstrual time. I do not abuse my children physically, but I do verbally, and I think that that can be almost as damaging, although I do try to explain to them why I behave the way I do, and apologize for it. The trouble begins as early as twelve to fourteen days after the beginning of the last period, and the first sign is a disturbance of sleep. I get violent dreams and often wake up at night. When it is time to get up, I feel as though I have had no rest at all. Then I become so tense I positively shake, and am so nervous and irritable that I am sorry for anyone who has to live with me. Quite often my heart starts to pound for no obvious reason, though I have not been running or doing heavy exercise. I feel listless and apathetic and often fall asleep during the day. On the other hand, the other half of the cycle I sleep perfectly soundly, and I am energetic, hard-working, and clear-headed. The onset of my period releases the tension, but triggers off headaches that fluctuate from day to day for a couple of days. I cry at the drop of a hat during all this time, and find it hard to deal with any problems objectively. Although I have been very depressed sometimes, I have never had a breakdown, thanks probably to good professional help. Apart from this misery, the rest of the month I am healthy, active, and very rarely ill.

Premenstrual tension, usually abbreviated as PMT, is only one aspect of PMS, which includes the bodily, physical, or somatic symptoms as well as the psychological ones. Some try to cope with it alone. A competent boutique manager wrote,

For many years I have managed to keep my PMT a secret, but increasingly I have found it more difficult to suppress. Friends have commented on unexpected changes in my behavior and totally irrational responses to situations. I feel desperate and helpless that I am no longer able to manage my PMT, but it has become a dominant factor in my life today. Normally, I am quite a positive and optimistic person.

The tension may come on quite suddenly, with an inability to relax and a general feeling of uptightness. One woman complained that when she was in this state she trembled so much that she had difficulty even threading a needle. Frequently, women are shy about mentioning premenstrual tension to their doctor, thinking that it is a common and minor complaint. Instead they complain of what is known by the medical profession as a "passport symptom"—a somatic symptom like a headache, backache, or flu, which they consider more acceptable. One mother wrote,

> When I go to the doctor I am always conscious that I am not physically ill, and so I do not want to tell him all my seemingly petty feelings. After all, one does not want to admit being a failure as a wife and mother.

Sometimes the tension reaches almost manic proportions, with such agitation and restless energy that the woman cannot calm down; she keeps walking up and down, or won't stop talking and repeats herself endlessly. One husband was upset because, as he said,

> It's no use trying to tell her to relax, she just keeps repeating herself and won't stop talking. New thoughts keep tumbling out. She accuses me of all sorts of things. She just goes on and on and on.

EFFECTS OF STRESS

Premenstrual tension, like all other symptoms of PMS, is always aggravated by other stress. None of us can be totally free from stress in our daily life. Work may be more demanding some days because co-workers are absent, or a friend or neighbor may be involved in an accident. The usual effect of these stresses will be an increase in premenstrual tension when the next menstruation approaches. On the other hand, good news will tend to ease the tension, and of course, a winning lottery ticket can be most beneficial in relieving premenstrual tension—though only for a month or two!

DEPRESSION

Depression may be so mild that the word *depression* is not used, or is even denied. For example, the woman may say that she is "fed up" or "feeling down," that she can't laugh easily and has difficulty smiling, or that the whole world is against her and nobody cares. Or the depression may range to the other extreme, with a black cloud hanging over everything, interfering with concentration, so that even simple tasks like reading or playing board games become impossible, and there is the ever-present possibility of suicide.

This risk of possible suicide should always be fully appreciated. One husband wrote describing his wife's depression:

I feel her life is at risk; she dreads these times so much it colors her whole life. She feels there is no hope.

And a mother described her twenty-year-old daughter's depression:

These occurrences are so regular that for years I have associated them with periods. But when she goes to her doctor, usually in a state of panic, she is either told to pull herself together or given tranquilizers. On at least three occasions she has taken the whole bottle and has had to have her stomach pumped. When she is in this state, she often becomes violent and smashes things or fights with her boyfriend. She may consume vast quantities of alcohol and then try to cut her wrists, always in the wrong direction. After the period, when she is herself, she is such a nice, kind, and good-natured person.

SUICIDE

A Washington, D.C., secretary ended her full description of premenstrual depression with the statement,

> The sad thing is that although suicidal thoughts cross my mind at this time, I am a very happy person ordinarily.

The MacKinnons, a husband-and-wife team of doctors, showed as long ago as 1956 that successful suicides predominated during the premenstruum. Studies of attempted suicides in hospitals in London and Delhi, and among the Samaritans in Los Angeles, have all confirmed that half of all women's attempts at suicide are made during the four days immediately before her period or the first four days of menstruation.

Although women make more suicide attempts than men, men succeed more frequently. This difference gradually disappears after the age of fifty. Dr. John Pollitt, speaking at the Royal Society of Medicine in 1976, suggested:

> Perhaps one reason for the female's lack of success is that the majority of attempts are made during the premenstrual phase or menstruation. Killing oneself is not easy; success requires careful planning. Women in the premenstrual phase show a marked tendency to be careless, thoughtless, unpunctual, forgetful, and absent-minded. This inefficiency at a time when they are more likely to try to end their lives may result in disproportionate failures.

Every suicidal gesture should be taken seriously. A sufferer's mood may deteriorate so suddenly just before or during menstruation that she may attempt suicide at a most unexpected moment. The attempt may end her life, even though it was only intended to be a cry for help, or it may result in permanent damage that is even harder to cope with than the premenstrual complaint. Drug overdoses may result in permanent liver or kidney damage, and if a woman throws herself in front of a car or jumps off a bridge, a scarred face or broken limbs will be ever-present reminders of the event that made her life so intolerable. One patient brought in diaries with a record of forty overdose attempts. Each one had required hospital admission and had occurred during her premenstruum, those four fateful days before menstruation.

Ellen, a twenty-four-year-old executive assistant, wrote,

> On December 6, realizing how dangerous the premenstrual effects were, I felt in great need of help. Unfortunately, my group meeting was during this time, and did not help me at all. After the meeting I rushed home, hid from my boyfriend whom I saw downtown, and intended again to overdose. Luckily, two friends arrived on the scene, and by the time they left it was all over and I had started to menstruate.

SELF-MUTILATION

When women, particularly young girls, are in deep despair, they may occasionally resort to self-mutilation by slashing their wrists, abdomen, neck, or face, or shaving their scalp or eyebrows. They may injure themselves severely, yet they apparently experience no pain; they appear to be anesthetized during the process. Self-mutilation is rare in men, and although it can occur in any woman, it appears to be most frequent among sufferers of PMS, so much so that when self-mutilation occurs, it is important to first eliminate the possibility of PMS before resorting to routine antidepressant therapy.

DEPRESSIVE ILLNESS

Depression can be an emotional reaction, such as we have when we hear of the death of a close friend or of other bad news, but it can also be an illness and affect bodily functions as well. The symptoms of a depressive illness are similar to those of premenstrual depression, but there are differences, one being the timing. In a typical depressive illness the symptoms are present day after day throughout the entire month and may last for weeks, months, or years. In premenstrual depression the symptoms do not last longer than fourteen days, for after menstruation the woman is her normal self. Another important difference is the marked irritability that accompanies premenstrual depression. A patient experiencing typical depression, on the other hand, may be too apathetic or lethargic to show any irritability, even on those occasions when it could be justified.

While problems with sleep are common in both premenstrual and typical depression, they differ in type. Although women with PMS may wake up during the night or early in the morning (and even get up to pass water), they yearn for sleep and don't tend to want to get out of bed until midday or later. Those with typical depression are more likely to wake in the early morning, when they get up to make a hot drink, have a good read, or possibly even do some housework.

There is also a difference in the appetites of those with the two different types of depression. Whereas women with typical depression lose their appetite and so lose weight, women with PMS tend to have a voracious appetite, with food cravings in the premenstruum, and they gain weight.

In typical depression there is an abysmal loss of sex interest, but on the contrary, especially among young adolescents, there may be a positive increase in libido in those with premenstrual depression. Premenstrual depression increases with age after twenty-six years and is common among single women.

	PMS Depression	*Depressive Illness*
Duration	14 days	weeks or years
Irritability	always present	may be absent
Sleep	yearning to stay in bed	early-morning waking
Appetite	increased	absent
Weight	gain	loss
Libido	may increase	absent

Depression is best thought of as a disease of loss, for there is a loss of happiness, interests, enthusiasm, memory, energy, sleep, and sexual arousal. One feels a loss of security and adequacy, and a loss of the powers of concentration, so that it becomes difficult to read a book or follow a television show. There is a loss of self-control accompanied by an inability to make decisions or to control one's tears, behavior, and appetite. There is a loss of insight and an inability to realize, in the case of premenstrual depression, that very shortly the symptoms will pass and there will be a return to normalcy.

TIREDNESS

"What worries me most is that I get so slow and stupid before my periods." This comment by a journalist is echoed by many who find the lethargy, exhaustion, and fatigue so difficult to cope with during the premenstruum. The "I-can't-be-bothered" attitude takes over and disrupts the program for the day, until in the end, "everything goes."

Frances, a thirty-two-year-old working mother, hated the tiredness most, and wrote,

> The worst and most worrying symptom is the feeling of apathy that descends on me. All physical and mental activity becomes a real effort and all I want to do is curl up in a corner away from everyone and all my responsibilities. I find it quite frightening that I cannot think clearly or quickly, and feel mentally dulled. These symptoms get increasingly worse, and a couple of days before a period I feel quite ill. The first day of a period I feel a bit headachy and tired, but then it is like a weight being lifted off me and for two weeks or so I feel really fine.

This tiredness may lead to withdrawal and a wish to hide, so aptly described by a secretary as follows:

A total withdrawal from all social contacts and withdrawing into myself. Despite living with friends, I often find myself not wanting to speak unless absolutely necessary, and often only manage one or two sentences.

Again, the tiredness may vary in severity. It can affect the typist who fills her wastebasket with typing errors, or the executive who feels unable to compose letters and stares all day at a blank sheet of paper. A mother of two boys, aged one and three, wrote,

When I feel bad I stay in bed all day. One day during my last vacation I felt so bad I couldn't bear to lift my sons or get them dressed, so the poor kids had to stay in bed the whole day. I just cried and told them how sorry I was that I couldn't help them at all. I'm afraid the little ones who have known me like this may grow up into disturbed children, but I promise you I'm quite normal at other times in my cycle.

One woman, not yet known to me, called for an appointment and when describing her tiredness, added,

I seem to be in a daze on those days. I can't do anything right—more than once I've crossed the road to go to the restroom and found myself in the Men's Room.

Others confessed,

Just before a period, for about ten days, a sleepiness takes me over and all I want to do is sit down and sleep, so that no housework or proper cooking gets done.

These are the "take-out" meal days, and "wash-up tomorrow" days.

It is premenstrual fatigue that is responsible for the drop in mental ability in the days before menstruation (discussed further in chapter 10).

IRRITABILITY

Those who are closest to a sufferer of premenstrual irritability are most affected by her short fuse and explosions over trivial matters. This usually includes not only the nearest but also the dearest—the husband or partner, children, and parents. As one woman said,

> Pity those around me when the least things upset me. I hate everyone, I shout and pick quarrels, and the whole world gets on my nerves.

Premenstrual irritability is more common in relationships. Partners naturally have problems trying to deal with their supersensitive, edgy, irrational, and agitated other half during these days of each cycle. Too many cases end up with visits to a marriage counselor or in divorce.

The following three excerpts from women's letters suggest that the husband often suffers as much as his wife:

> I have been suffering from premenstrual tension for some years now, and recently it came to its height. I was in my usual depressed state and, being angry, didn't know what to do with myself, just lost my temper for the thousandth time and I kicked in the door and required forty stitches in my leg. My husband is at his wits' end. He doesn't know what to do with me, not knowing what I'm going to do next, and is ready to leave me after being married only eighteen months. I keep telling him that I'll be good the next time, but I never am and just can't control myself.

> Last Saturday I deliberately smashed all the dishes after clearing the table. I started menstruating in the evening.

My family doctor puts it down to my Irish temper. I get so depressed, hateful, and tired; I stay in bed and shout, and I could go on and on like this. It is my husband who asked me to write for help.

At thirty-two, there is very little hope for me except, perhaps, menopause. I have a history of suicide attempts, child- and husband-beating, and many fights with a long-suffering doctor, who has been accused by me of many crimes, neglect and attempted manslaughter among them. At my worst I have taken many prescribed antidepressants in massive overdoses.

If one sees a patient shortly after an aggressive outburst like those just described, it is sometimes possible to get full details about the time at which food was eaten during the day. It is a common finding that the irritability is always worse when, in addition to premenstrual tension, there has been a long interval since the last meal, causing the blood sugar level to fall (see the discussion of blood sugar levels in chapter 24). When patients are asked at what time of day their irritability increases, it is usually in the late morning if breakfast has been missed, or when preparing the evening meal or waiting for the husband if he is later than usual. Often the woman has only had a sandwich, or just cheese and an apple at midday, and has eaten nothing else in anticipation of the evening meal.

Sudden explosive outbursts of irritability or aggression can usually be helped by ensuring that regular small meals are taken at intervals of three hours. In two recent cases of murder and one of infanticide, it was found that the perpetrators had not eaten for nine hours.

CONFUSION

At the height of the premenstrual tension there may be true confusion and memory loss, so that the woman is unaware of her actions or surroundings. Indeed, she may bitterly deny her

actions, for she has no memory of them. The following notes
made by a patient show how extreme the confusion may be,
and how it may well represent temporary insanity:

> From July 4th onward, severe depression with secretive
> confusion. On the 7th I planned to kill my mother and
> myself. I wrote suicide notes to all concerned and took
> certain prescribed drugs that I thought would work. I do
> not know whether I would have done it, as my friend,
> with whom I have a good relationship, discovered them
> and flushed them down the toilet. It took quite a few days
> before I realized how bizarre the whole episode was. The
> loss of appetite, need for alcohol, aggression, lack of
> interest, and swollen glands continued until menstrua-
> tion started on the 9th. These notes are written on the
> 18th, when my mind is clear.

It is not surprising that premenstrual tension, with its
irritability and confusion, frequently leads to problems with
the law. There are those cases of aggression where, in a sudden fit of temper, a woman makes an unjustified assault on
her neighbor or boss, or violently attacks a police officer.
There are cases of baby battering, husband beating, and homicide. Becoming drunk and disorderly when under the influence of alcohol or drugs may also lead to charges. In France it
is recognized that premenstrual tension may become so acute
and so violent that it may be classified as temporary insanity
in courts of law.

My British survey, in 1961, of 156 newly incarcerated
women prisoners revealed that half had committed their crime
during the paramenstruum (the last four days before menstruation and the first four days of menstruation), and that PMS
was present in two-thirds of these women. Theft was the most
common crime, with 56 percent of incidents committed during the paramenstruum, while the alcoholics charged with
being drunk and disorderly were a close second at 54 percent.

In the same women's prison twenty years later, two psychiatrists, Dr. D'Orban and Joy Dalton (no relation to the authors), confirmed these findings in relation to crimes of violence, finding that 44 percent of the criminals had committed their offense during the paramenstruum and 34 percent suffered from PMS.

The Paris police noticed early in this century that 84 percent of violent crimes committed by women had been committed during the premenstruum or menstruation. This was confirmed by a similar study in New York, which showed that 62 percent of violent crimes were committed during the premenstruum.

Dr. Morton and his colleagues, working in Westfield State Prison, Bedford Hills, New York, showed that it was worthwhile treating the inmates of prisons and reformatories if they suffered from PMS. He found that treatment resulted in an increased work output, a decrease in punishment for disobeying rules, and an increase in general morale.

In fact, this question should be asked: What benefit will a woman gain from a prison sentence or fine if she is unable to control her premenstrual irritability or confusion? Most prisoners with PMS, if untreated, usually serve their full sentences without remission for good conduct, because too often their symptoms get the better of them each premenstruum and cause further problems, with the inevitable loss of privileges.

This chapter has dealt with symptoms in general and the psychological symptoms of PMS in detail; the next chapter discusses the physical PMS symptoms, which are invariably also present.

5

❧

Physical Symptoms of PMS

PMS is a hormonal disease in which hormones (progesterone) are carried in the blood and passed into target cells, which have special hormone (progesterone) receptors to carry the molecules into the nucleus (chapter 6). Not only the brain cells, which have progesterone receptors, but also numerous other cells around the body can be affected by a failure of progesterone receptors and thus cause symptoms. These physical, or bodily, symptoms vary according to the usual function of the cells. Thus, whereas progesterone is used by the brain cells to control emotions, in the bones it is used to build new bone cells. It is relatively rare to find women with PMS who have only psychological symptoms. While it is impossible to list all the possible symptoms, the most common ones are discussed in the following sections (Figure 7). Headache heads the list as the most common physical symptom of PMS.

HEADACHES

Many women, looking for a good reason, might be tempted to claim that their particular variety of headache comes only at period time. Undoubtedly, menstruation is the most frequent time for migraine attacks in women. This can be seen in Figure

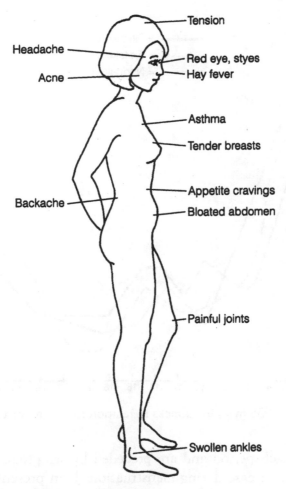

Figure 7 Common symptoms of PMS

8, in which the times of 935 migraine attacks are shown in relation to the days of the menstrual cycle.

Those who can produce a three-month record showing a regular and definite relationship of their headache to menstruation have a much better chance of obtaining relief through appropriate PMS treatment. In Figure 9 we can see that Isobel's headaches last between seven and ten days

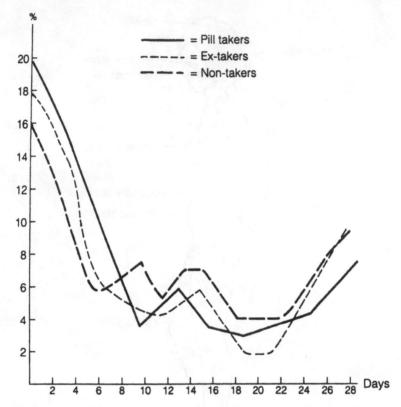

Figure 8   935 migraine attacks in relation to the menstrual cycle

before each period and are preceded by symptoms of tension, which ease during menstruation. Joan presents a different picture: her headaches last only one or two days and there is no premenstrual tension, but the headaches all tend to come around the time of menstruation. Kathleen seems to have headaches every ten or twelve days; occasionally they coincide with menstruation, but often they appear at any time. It is unlikely that Kathleen will benefit from hormonal treatment.

Generally, the monthly headaches that are likely to benefit from treatment with specific hormones such as progesterone are those that show a definite relationship to menstruation in

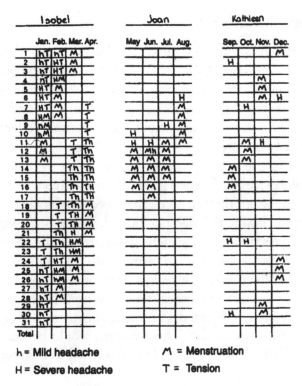

h = Mild headache   M = Menstruation

H = Severe headache   T = Tension

Figure 9   Headaches in relation to menstruation

a three-month record and have the characteristics of PMS discussed in chapter 2. Women with these headaches are likely to be free from headaches after the fourth month of pregnancy, and they may well look back to the later months of pregnancy as the only time in their life when they knew what that freedom was like. Unfortunately, these same women are also likely to say that immediately after their pregnancy the headaches returned and were worse than ever.

The majority of these women are also likely to find that after the menopause most of these problems come to an end.

The three common types of headaches related to menstruation are sinus or vacuum headaches, tension headaches, and migraines.

Vacuum Headaches

It is better to speak of vacuum headaches rather than sinus headaches, as the latter are likely to be confused with headaches resulting from true sinusitis, which is caused by infected material getting lodged in the sinuses, and are not likely to be related to menstruation. Vacuum headaches, on the other hand, are caused by the swelling of the cells at the entrance to the sinus, which block the entry so that stale air accumulates inside. Women generally know that a headache is on the way when their nasal passages become blocked and it is difficult to breathe through one nostril. There is tenderness or pressure over the sinuses, which are situated in the cheekbones and over the eyes. The resulting pain worsens when the woman bends over and may last from one to seven days. In addition, there may be other signs of waterlogging, such as a gain in weight, a bloated abdomen, shortness of breath, or swollen ankles or fingers. These women would be wise to follow the Three-Hourly Starch Diet discussed in chapter 24.

Tension Headaches

Tension headaches usually have a slow onset, so that a woman who is trying to chart her symptoms may be uncertain whether the pain in her head is bad enough to call a headache. A tension headache usually starts after symptoms of premenstrual tension—irritability, tiredness, or depression—and eases off gradually during the course of menstruation. The pain from tension headaches has been described as "a steel band enclosing my head" or "like a heavy weight on top of my head" (see Figure 10). These women will find that the usual analgesics, such as aspirin or paracetamol, will give relief for only about four hours—then the headache returns and the analgesic must be repeated. Treatment with progesterone (see chapter 25) is most valuable for this type of headache, and it has the added advantage of relieving the other symptoms of PMS.

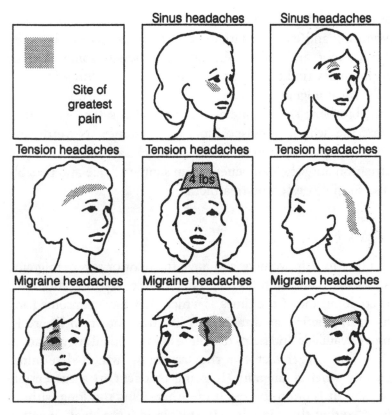

Figure 10   Sites of greatest pain in menstrual headaches

Migraines

Doctors like to divide migraines into two varieties: the classic and the common. In the classic variety the patient has a warning, or "aura," that lasts for about twenty minutes before the onset of a severe headache. This aura may take the form of sudden flashes of lights, brightly colored stars and stripes, or a patch of blindness; or there may be a sensation of pins and needles in the tongue, the side of the face, or the hands and legs. Many people suffer from both classic and common migraines at different times over the years. Common migraines have no aura and begin gradually, increasing in severity. Both migraines may be accompanied by nausea or vomiting and extreme fatigue, and they usually last between twenty-four and forty-eight hours, although some unlucky women may find that their migraines last even longer.

Most migraine sufferers have a family history, with a parent, brothers, sisters, uncles, or aunts also suffering, so they start life with a predisposition to migraines. Nevertheless, there are those among them whose attacks are related to menstruation and who can benefit from simple advice and possibly also from progesterone treatment.

Attack Form

In order to help women who have frequent or severe migraine attacks, it is helpful to have full details of everything they have been doing and of the times at which they have consumed any food. In practice, an attack form like that shown in Figure 11 proves valuable and helps to isolate an individual trigger factor.

The trigger factor is the last straw, which determines exactly when a migraine is going to occur in a susceptible woman. It is often the result of either going too long without food, so that there is a drop in the blood sugar level, or eating foods to which the sufferer is sensitive.

When women are asked what sort of things start a migraine attack, they often mention travel, going to the movies, or working hard for several days for a special event, like a garage sale, a wedding, or a big party. If the attack forms have been carefully filled in, it is usually easy to spot if the migraine has been caused by too long an interval without food. Generally speaking, five hours between meals is a good length of time for most women leading a normal, energetic life, but a three-hour interval between meals is advised for those suffering from PMS (see pages 223–224). An overnight interval of thirteen hours is usually considered the limit. After this length of time, susceptible women, probably those born with the tendency to get migraines, will find they develop a headache. This

Name ....   Date ....
                                            Day of week ....
                                            Time of onset ....
                                            Duration ....
Day of cycle ....   Days before next menstruation .....

During the 24 hours *before* an attack:

(1) Did you have any special worry, overwork, or shock?

(2) What had you done during the day:
      Normal work?
      Unusual activity?
      Extra tired?

(3) What food had you eaten and when?

      Breakfast ....   Time ....
      ....
      Mid-morning ....   Time ....
      ....
      Lunch ....   Time ....
      ....
      Mid-afternoon ....   Time ....
      ....
      Supper ....   Time ....
      ....
      Evening ....   Time ....
      ....
      Bedtime ....   Time ....
      ....

Figure 11   An attack form useful for isolating trigger factors
in migraine

explains why travel often causes a headache: with frequent
interruptions and long distances traveled, meals are often
delayed longer than usual. Similarly, if one is busy with preparations for special events, food may easily be forgotten. And if
you are giving the party, how easy it is to ensure that your guests
have plenty while forgetting to eat anything yourself.

   One must also consider not only the interval between
meals but also the amount of energy expended during the interval. The more energy that is used, the quicker the blood sugar
level falls. Overnight fasting is often the cause of a migraine

attack on waking, and there are those migraine sufferers who say they cannot sleep late on holidays or weekends because they wake up with a headache. Migraines are also likely to occur when some energetic sport or a brisk walk follows an evening meal and no further food is taken before going to bed.

An example of this was noted in a receptionist who was an avid skater and normally had her evening meal at 6:30 P.M. On Thursday evenings she would go to the rink for three hours of energetic recreation, but she would have no food after the evening meal. Every four or five weeks, she would wake with a migraine on Friday mornings. The attacks occurred during the paramenstruum but were triggered by the long interval without food and the energetic skating.

Full information about the effect of a drop in blood sugar levels is given on pages 223–224. If the attack forms show that the woman has gone without food for too long or has been too energetic for the amount of food she has consumed, a sudden drop in blood sugar may have triggered the attack. In that case the treatment is obvious: avoid fasting, and remember to have an extra cookie with your morning and afternoon coffee or tea. Remember, too, that proteins such as meat, fish, and eggs will keep the blood sugar up longer, while candy will cause a short, sharp rise in blood sugar level followed by a quick drop, and thus provide only a temporary benefit.

Foods Causing Migraine

Women whose migraine attacks are not caused by fasting may find that they are sensitive to certain foods, the most common of which are cheese, chocolate, alcohol, and citrus fruits. A few are sensitive to ripe bananas, pork, onions, fish, or gluten. In these cases the migraine attacks do not occur immediately after the specific food has been eaten, but some twelve to thirty-six hours later. This is because the attack occurs not when the food is digested in the stomach but later, when it is broken down in the liver by the action of the special chemicals known as enzymes. Apparently, if one particular enzyme is not present, a wrong chemical action occurs, releasing substances capable of opening wide the blood vessels of the brain. These substances are known as *vasodilating amines*. Two common ones are tyramine, which is present in cheese, and phenylethylamine, which is present in alcohol and chocolate; but there are other vasodilating amines that can be formed by the wrong breakdown of everyday foods. Some women's sensitivity to vasodilating amines may be increased during the paramenstruum, so that although they are able to take small amounts of cheese, for example, after menstruation, if they eat cheese as menstruation approaches or during menstruation, even a minute amount is sufficient to provoke an attack. Women who fall into this category should try to avoid the foods to which they are sensitive, remembering always that these sensitivities vary from person to person. Foods that cause attacks in one individual will not necessarily cause attacks in another migraine sufferer.

One theory of sensitivity suggests that when the individual's sensitive food is processed through the liver it leaves behind a small amount of toxin, say 5 percent, which is not enough to cause trouble, but after the person has had the sensitive food on several occasions the toxin may have risen to 95 percent. So then it will take only a very small amount of the sensitive food to produce an attack. These sensitive foods will show up when several attack forms are studied.

However, as mentioned earlier, there are often other members of the family who also suffer from migraines, so it may be worthwhile having a "gathering of the clan" at which all blood relations who suffer from migraine can exchange ideas. Often, they may find a common food to which all family members are sensitive. A London family, in which the grandmother, mother, and son all had problems with tomatoes, was surprised to find the same allergy to tomatoes present in the mother's nephew in Alaska and her niece in Argentina.

Those who are sensitive to cheese will be happy to learn that tyramine is not present in cream cheese or cottage cheese, but develops only when a cheese matures, so among the particular cheeses to be avoided are Stilton, cheddar, Parmesan, and processed cheeses. However, they should be aware that mature cheese is often hidden in quiches, Mornay sauce, and Italian dishes.

Red wine, sherry, port, and champagne are probably the worst alcohols for causing migraines, but it is often possible to take a single glass of white wine with food without any after-effects. It is also worth considering the difference between grape and grain alcohols, for more people are sensitive to grape alcohols than to grain alcohols like beer, vodka, and whiskey.

Chocolate is often added to rich fruit cakes or finger cakes to give a good color, and to coffee dishes to increase the flavor, so those who are sensitive to chocolate should be on their guard. Plain dark chocolate is more likely to provoke an attack than milk chocolate. It is very easy for those sensitive to citrus fruits to forget that this category also includes mandarins and tangerines.

WATER RETENTION

The mechanism that causes water retention in the premenstruum is discussed on page 57. The effects of water retention can be general, such as weight gain and bloatedness, as well as localized, such as sties, joint pains, or uveitis. Any tissues of the body may be affected, the actual site varying with individuals, often with a family sensitivity to one area. The most common sign of water being retained in the body is an increase in weight, which generally averages four to seven pounds (see Figure 12) but can be even more, as much as ten to twelve pounds.

The normal weight is that which is taken during the postmenstruum, and gains and losses of up to five pounds are usually considered within normal limits for women. Dr. William Thomas of Chicago documented a case of one woman who gained between twelve and fourteen pounds each premenstruum, and then lost it with an excessive output of nine pints of urine on the first day of menstruation, the excessive urine

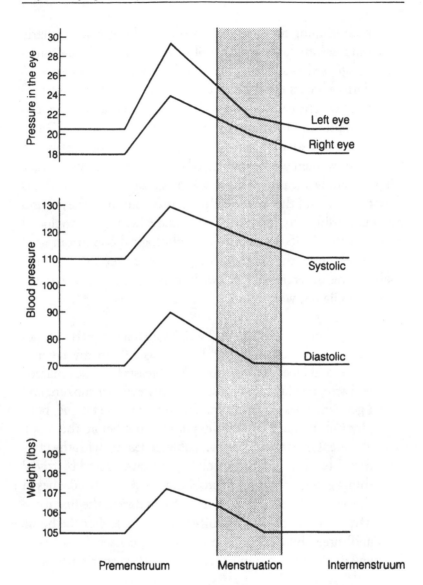

Figure 12   Fluctuations in weight, blood pressure, and pressure in the eye during the menstrual cycle of a PMS sufferer

output continuing for the next few days. Those who regularly gain and lose very large amounts of water periodically are sometimes diagnosed as suffering from cyclical idiopathic edema.

Early workers on PMS believed that the amount of premenstrual weight gain was an index of the severity of premenstrual symptoms, but this is definitely not the case. Dr. Bruce and Professor Russell of Maudsley Hospital, London, examined thirty-four women who complained of premenstrual symptoms. They carefully measured their weights, the amount of fluids they took in, and the amount they passed out, and they found no relationship. In fact, the researchers wrongly concluded from this that PMS was a purely psychological condition.

Apart from the gain in weight, water retention shows itself in the different tissues, with varying effects, as experienced by Gladys, who wrote,

> The pattern of a five-pound weight increase at period times makes me so bloated that I no longer fit in my favorite slacks, and I feel ready to burst. My breasts become enlarged and sore, needing a larger size bra, my eyes get sunken, and I get dark rings under them. There is extreme fatigue, both physical, so that I can hardly put one foot before the other, and mental, so that I feel incapable of dealing with the children I teach. I get into black depressions, caused by trivial things going wrong. I get throbbing and severe headaches in the week before my period, and always during the first three days of bleeding. I work a full-time job, look after the home and three children, and go to evening classes. I also paint and do flower arranging . . . so you see I do try to fight it.

The extra water in the tissues can cause ankles and fingers to swell, so that shoes have to be discarded and rings removed. There may be swelling of the gums, so dentures no longer fit. The skin coarsens and becomes blotchy, contact lenses won't fit, and the hair becomes stringy. One model, who refused to accept work during the premenstruum, said,

I look my very worst—my skin won't take make-up, my
face goes stiff, and I can't move gracefully with those
extra pounds of weight!

The exact place where the water accumulates varies in different women and at different times in their life. The most severe
symptoms result from water accumulating in a small area that
does not allow for stretching, such as the labyrinth of the inner
ear, which causes dizziness; the eyeball, causing raised pressure
inside the eye and severe pain; and inside the unyielding, bony
skull, causing headaches. The sinuses are air spaces within the
bones of the face where air enters through a small entrance that
is lined with cells of the mucus membrane. When these are
engorged and swollen, the entrance to the sinus is blocked, causing stale air to accumulate and resulting in sinus headaches or
"vacuum headaches." Water can also accumulate in the discs
between the vertebrae of the spine, causing backaches.

Sometimes there is a widespread distribution of the extra
water, which produces vague symptoms in the muscles, joints,
and soft tissues, causing generalized rheumatic pains, abdominal bloating, and heaviness. The water is always in the cells or
in the fluid between the cells, never free, although one patient
imagined she could hear the water "splashing inside her
abdomen," and another described how her abdomen was "gur-
gling and swimming in water." When the extra water accumulates in the fat and subcutaneous tissues, there can be an
appreciable gain in weight, without any other complaints.
This is most likely to happen in obese women. One speaker at
a medical lecture observed, tongue-in-cheek, that "Today, no
woman suffers from obesity, only from water retention."

Locating the Water

The actual sites where the cells become swollen may vary from
time to time, depending on factors such as anatomical abnormality, heredity, injury, and infection. Thus, a premenstrual

sinus headache is more likely to occur in a woman whose nose cartilage is bent. Water is readily attracted to cells that have recently been injured or infected, so that after a fracture of the leg or arm it is common to notice premenstrual swelling there for some months. If water retention occurs during the pre-menstruum in someone who has recently had pneumonia, it may cause a return of the cough or breathlessness.

This water retention is often blamed for the depression and other symptoms that accompany it. Helen, a twenty-seven-year-old accountant, wrote,

> I start to get tender, swollen breasts, usually fourteen days (ovulation?) before the beginning of menstruation, and I gain several pounds in weight. This makes me depressed and bad-tempered, and when you feel like that you can't help getting annoyed with everyone around you.

Many of the symptoms of water retention are typically worse in the early morning, often waking the patient from her sleep. This is especially so with migraines, with the acute pain in the eyeball that mimics glaucoma, and with asthma, when there is swelling of the lining cells of the small tubes of the lung. A feeling of pins and needles, and perhaps numbness of the fingers, may awaken some people. This is because the nerve passes from the arm through a narrow, bony tunnel at the wrist, and when the surrounding cells are swollen and waterlogged, this nerve becomes constricted. This odd sensation is called carpal tunnel syndrome. If severe, it can be relieved by a simple operation designed to decompress the trapped nerve.

Many drugs are available nowadays that help to increase the amount of urine passed, and these would seem to be a simple answer to the problem of water retention. Unfortunately, the problem is not quite so simple. Although these drugs, or diuretics, can get rid of water, extra water forms again quickly. It is rather like bailing water from a boat with a hole in it: it is better to close up the hole and prevent further water from entering than to just keep bailing. And as bailers get tired, so do the water tablets, and the cells tend to lose their elasticity. The temptation then is to use stronger and stronger drugs to get rid of more and more water. When diuretics were first introduced, they tended to cause both water and potassium to pass out of the body in the urine. The depletion of potassium caused increased tiredness and weakness of the limbs. There is now a new class of potassium-sparing diuretics that do not upset the potassium level, and these should be the first choice if diuretics are really needed to alleviate symptoms of PMS.

Patients who have received diuretics continually for many years tend to become dehydrated. These patients complain strongly, within a day or two, of feeling bloated if the diuretics are stopped suddenly. They need to gradually taper off their diuretics, using them on alternate days, starting immediately in the postmenstruum. After a month or two it may be possible to decrease the dose to every third or fourth day, until they are used only when the weight gain is really marked.

BREAST SORENESS

Complaints of breast soreness with enlarged and tender nipples are common in PMS. Frequently, women who experience this fear it may be a sign of breast cancer. It is definitely not related to cancer in any way. What is happening is that the breast tissue is getting ready in the event that, following ovulation, a pregnancy will occur, and the breasts will be needed for breast-feeding. It must be emphasized that not all cases of breast tenderness are due to PMS—only those cases where cyclical soreness is present in the premenstruum with complete absence of pain after menstruation. A menstrual chart completed daily will quickly show whether the symptom is present daily, cyclically, or only at ovulation. Breast swelling that is present throughout the month but more marked in the paramenstruum may be caused by increased output of the hormone *prolactin* from the pituitary gland. It is possible to measure the blood prolactin level, and if this is high, treatment with bromocriptine may help. It must not be forgotten that breasts are sexually charged areas, and when a woman is having problems in her sex life, her breasts may become more sensitive. Nipple sensitivity, as opposed to breast tenderness, may also result from taking vitamin B-6, even at low doses, over a long period.

ASTHMA

Premenstrual asthma appears to be caused by water retention in the cells lining the smaller tubes of the lung, which become swollen and prevent the free entry of air into the minute air sacs. Thus the cause is not necessarily allergic. In fact, these patients may not respond to sodium cromoglycate (Intal) inhalers or steroids, as do those whose asthma has a definite allergic basis. Premenstrual asthma is particularly common in women in the thirties and forties, and it often starts or increases with estrogen therapy at menopause. Heavy smokers are particularly at risk. Usually, the women will say that their attacks are brought on by tension and stress, but that may be because they have not yet connected them to PMS. In the special asthma clinics in hospitals it is usual for about one-third of all women of childbearing age to have menstrually related asthma. Two patients, aged eighteen (see *Sara*, pages 255–256) and forty-two, who were treated at the PMS Clinic at the University College Hospital, London, had a record of over twenty admissions to intensive care units for acute asthma. Finally, an alert nurse noticed that their attacks always occurred premenstrually. Both have since become free from asthma after receiving progesterone treatment.

EPILEPSY

One of the most satisfying experiences for a doctor is to be able to diagnose and treat a woman with premenstrual epilepsy. She can be treated with progesterone and taken off all anticonvulsant tablets, with their many unpleasant side effects. Furthermore, in Britain, if a person is not taking anticonvulsant drugs and has been three years without an epileptic seizure, she has the joy of having her driver's license restored.

Premenstrual epilepsy is often a culminating symptom, which follows gradually increasing tension and headache, so these patients do have a warning that an attack is imminent. There may also be marked weight gain, though this is not always the case. Often the final trigger factor that precipitates the attack is a long interval without food.

Laura, twenty-eight years old, with one child, left for her vacation having had only a light breakfast at 8:00 A.M. Her husband drove some three hundred miles, stopping only to ask for directions. When she arrived at her hotel she had a nasty headache, and while she was unpacking, at about 5:00 P.M., she had an epileptic seizure. She started menstruating the next day. She later agreed that there had been mounting tension during the previous week, which she had attributed to trying to finish all the necessary jobs in time for her vacation. (See *Laura*, page 256.)

The charts of two other epileptic patients, Margaret (see page 255) and Nancy, are shown in Figure 13. Both responded completely to progesterone treatment and both had their driver's licenses restored.

OTHER PHYSICAL SYMPTOMS

Rhinitis, or *hay fever*, may be mistaken for the common cold. It is usual to hear women in April saying, "You know, this is the fourth cold I've had since Christmas," when in fact it is premenstrual rhinitis occurring along with their fourth menstruation since Christmas. The rhinitis is caused by extra water, which in turn causes the swelling of the cells of the nasal passages. Once it is recognized as a premenstrual symptom, there is no need to prescribe antihistamines or antibiotics. If the swelling of the cells occurs a little lower down in the larynx it

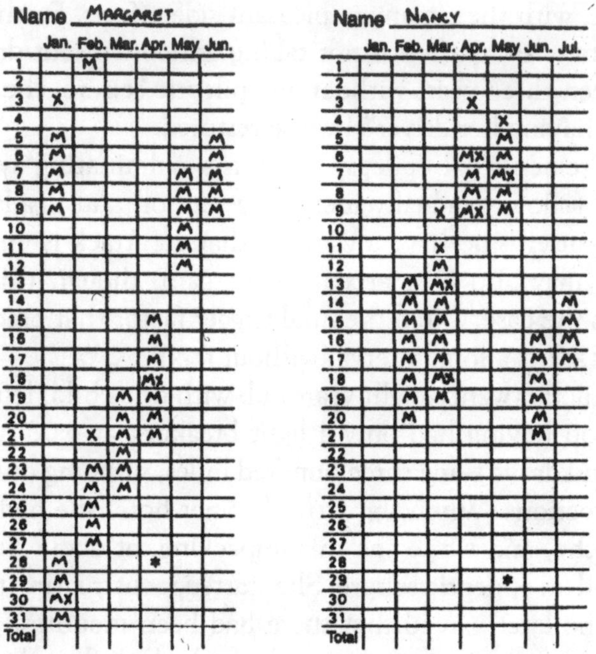

Name __MARGARET__

	Jan.	Feb.	Mar.	Apr.	May	Jun.
1		M				
2						
3	X					
4						
5	M					M
6	M					M
7	M				M	M
8	M				M	M
9	M				M	M
10					M	
11					M	
12					M	
13						
14						
15				M		
16				M		
17				M		
18				MX		
19			M	M		
20			M	M		
21		X	M	M		
22			M			
23		M	M			
24		M	M			
25		M				
26		M				
27		M				
28	M			*		
29	M					
30	MX					
31	M					
Total						

Margaret is 27 yrs old with 2 children, onset after 1st pregnancy

Name __NANCY__

	Jan.	Feb.	Mar.	Apr.	May	Jun.	Jul.
1							
2							
3			X				
4				X			
5				M			
6			MX	M			
7				M	MX		
8				M	M		
9			X	MX	M		
10							
11		X					
12		M					
13	M	MX					
14	M	M					M
15	M	M					M
16	M	M			M		M
17	M	M			M		M
18	M	MX			M		
19	M	M			M		
20	M				M		
21					M		
22							
23							
24							
25							
26							
27							
28							
29					*		
30							
31							
Total							

Nancy is 28 yrs old, onset at puberty

M = menstruation
x = epileptic attack
* = progesterone treatment started

Figure 13   Charts of two patients with premenstrual epilepsy

can cause hoarseness, which is a special nuisance to singers. One opera singer carefully arranged her singing engagements to avoid her premenstruum. Another remarked that during the premenstruum the quality of her voice changed, and she was unable to reach the high notes. This was corrected by progesterone therapy.

The *loss of the sense of smell* is probably more common than generally appreciated. It is caused by extra water accumulating in the cells that are responsible for the sense of smell. The manufacturer of a special brand of antiperspirant/deodorant noticed that women tended to change their brand every three or four weeks, complaining that it had ceased to function effectively. Market research showed that the dissatisfaction was due to a premenstrual increase in perspiration and vaginal discharge, and a diminishing ability to smell the reassuring perfume of the antiperspirant/deodorant product. This led women to believe that the product had lost its effectiveness.

Dizziness or *vertigo* is a common premenstrual complaint: in some surveys it occurred in one-third of all PMS sufferers. It is most frequent among those who have had children and are approaching menopause. The dizziness gets worse if the woman bends over, and it may accompany a headache. The probable cause is excess fluid in the labyrinth of the ear, which is responsible for balance.

Fainting is common just before menstruation and is most likely to occur when there has been a long interval without food, or prolonged standing. In England fainting is common among teenage schoolgirls who have missed their breakfast and have to stand for a long time at the early-morning school assembly.

Cystitis and *urethritis* are common symptoms during the premenstruum and may be caused by the increase in vaginal discharge and generalized pelvic congestion.

Joint and muscle pains may come back each month just before menstruation, last only a few days, and then disappear without treatment. There may also be stiffness on waking in the morning, although this disappears within the hour. Localized swelling of the cells, or failure of muscle relaxation during the time of premenstrual tension, probably causes the pain. The water retention that accompanies many of these symptoms led to the mistaken theory that PMS was caused by water retention and could therefore be corrected by diuretics. The effect of such treatment has already been discussed (see page 60).

There are many factors responsible for the formation of *varicose veins*, including a tendency within the family. However, when they first begin to appear they may be visible only in the premenstruum, and later they may be painful only at this time of the cycle. Cynics usually say you should have chosen your parents more carefully.

Boils, sties, and *acne* are all common skin lesions, which frequently recur each cycle just before menstruation. Acne is perhaps a special case. It is caused by the grease (or sebum) produced by the sebaceous glands in the skin being too thick and plentiful. This grease is excreted through the pores of the skin. If the grease is too thick, it blocks the pores and causes acne. The skin only starts making grease, or sebum, at puberty, so in the first few years of its production often there is either too much, or it is too thick or too thin. Gradually, the body learns to make the right amount. Estrogen helps to slow down the production of grease, so acne often returns at the time of falling estrogen levels, such as at ovulation and before menstruation. This also explains why acne usually improves during pregnancy when there is plenty of estrogen and also in some women on the high-dosage estrogen pill.

Conjunctivitis or *red eye* may return each month due to causes other than infection. It is interesting that the association of conjunctivitis with menstruation was known as long ago as the sixteenth century.

Glaucoma is caused by raised pressure within the eyeball. This may be due to a narrowing of the opening through which the circulating fluid in the eyeball drains. It is not surprising to find that when there is water retention during the premenstruum, there may be an excess accumulation of fluid within the eye, and also difficulty in draining it away (see Figure 14). When this happens, the pressure within the eye is raised, which becomes very painful and, by pressure on the optic nerve, may interfere with sight. A survey of patients of menstruating age with closed-angle glaucoma (where the draining opening is blocked) at the Institute of Ophthalmology in London revealed that 89 percent suffered from PMS. A rise in intraocular levels is common regardless of the initial level (Figure 14).

Uveitis and *iritis* are two other troublesome eye conditions that tend to flare up premenstrually and respond to progesterone treatment.

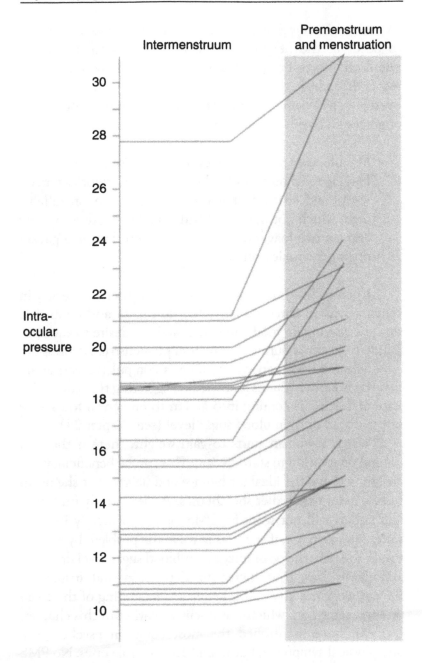

Figure 14   Menstrual rise in intraocular pressure (131 readings)

Capricious appetite, food cravings, and *binges* are well known to occur at the height of premenstrual tension and water retention. However great her self-control may be during the rest of the month, there come those days when a woman is just overtaken by a demon and eats enough for a week in one meal, or gorges on sweets. Olive wrote,

> My life swings between cycles of feasting and fasting. Having lived on a careful diet of only 750 calories for two weeks and losing four pounds, I had an uncontrollable urge, which got me out of bed. I raided Mother's pantry and ate two loaves of bread with peanut butter, a packet of ginger cookies, and some apple pie.

Doctors Smith and Sauder from McMaster University in Canada studied three hundred female nurses and confirmed that the craving for food and sweets and the desire to eat compulsively occurred during the times of premenstrual depression.

The foods chosen when there is compulsive eating are invariably carbohydrates and sweets, suggesting that the body's natural defense is coming into action to prevent a too severe or prolonged drop in blood sugar level (see chapter 24).

When a woman starts to gain weight, there is the very natural temptation to start dieting. This can be beneficial if her weight is above the ideal for her age and height, but she needs to be careful which diet she chooses. A diet of only fruit juice and liquids will not work for PMS, as it will merely increase water retention. Or, if she tries to solve the problem by missing meals, she risks the possibility of her blood sugar level dropping abnormally low, thus increasing depression and irritability. Recent work has given us a better understanding of the cause of water retention, which was discussed earlier in this chapter.

We have mentioned the most common psychological and physical symptoms, but not all 150 possible ones. No PMS sufferer will experience only one symptom, but fortunately, no individual suffers from them all.

6

PMS Is a Hormonal Disease

A woman is born with two ovaries containing thousands of immature egg cells. Each month, in response to a message from the pituitary gland at the base of the brain, one of the unripe egg cells develops inside a tiny microscopic ring of cells, which gradually increases to form a little balloon or cyst called the Graafian follicle. These cells make the menstrual hormone *estrogen*, about which we will be hearing more later. When the little egg cell is fully developed it appears as a blister on the surface of the ovary, and when it receives a further message from the pituitary gland it bursts and releases the mature egg cell. This is known as *ovulation*. This process can be seen with ultrasound imaging, which allows one to watch the tiny cyst growing day by day and suddenly bursting, or rather disappearing, from view.

The egg cell makes its way down a fallopian tube to the womb, a journey that takes about fourteen days. Meanwhile, the yellow scar tissue left behind when the blister bursts fills up with new cells that produce the second important menstrual hormone, *progesterone*.

PROGESTERONE, THE PREGNANCY HORMONE

The progesterone acts on the lining of the womb to turn it into a soft, spongy layer in which the fertilized egg cell can embed itself if a pregnancy occurs. During intercourse, millions of male sperm are projected into the vagina and journey through the womb up into one of the fallopian tubes in an attempt to fertilize the egg cell, so that conception will occur and pregnancy can begin. The fertilized egg passes into the womb and becomes embedded in the new soft lining, where it develops into a baby. Following successful fertilization, progesterone will continue to be produced by the ovary for about three months, and by the placenta from two months until the birth. Progesterone is essential for the growing fetus and to protect the developing baby from being rejected by the mother's womb. However, if the egg cell has not been fertilized, the production of progesterone begins to fall. About fourteen days after ovulation, the soft, spongy lining of the womb, which is then not needed, disintegrates and is shed, together with the unfertilized egg cell. This is menstruation, which represents a failed pregnancy.

PHASES OF THE MENSTRUAL CYCLE

Although a normal menstrual cycle may vary from twenty-one to thirty-five days, it is easiest when discussing the phases of the menstrual cycle to consider a cycle of twenty-eight days. There are seven phases of the menstrual cycle that all have different levels of hormones circulating in the blood. A diagram of the relative timing of the four menstrual hormones is shown in Figure 15, and for comparison the steady daily levels of male hormones are shown in Figure 16.

The seven phases are as follows:

Days 1– 4   *Menstruation,* low estrogen with rise of follicle-stimulating hormone (FSH)

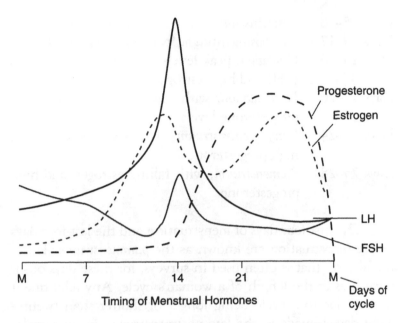

Figure 15   Relative hormone levels in the menstrual cycle

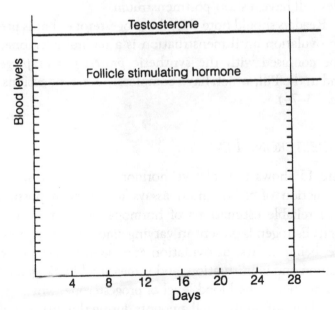

Figure 16   Male hormone levels during a month

Days 5– 8   *Postmenstruum*, rising estrogen levels

Days 9–12   *Late postmenstruum*, peak estrogen levels

Days 13–16   *Ovulation*, peak levels of luteinizing hormones (LH) and high estrogen

Days 17–20   *Postovulation*, with lower estrogen and rising progesterone levels

Days 21–24   *Early premenstruum*, with high estrogen and high progesterone

Days 25–28   *Premenstruum*, with falling estrogen and high progesterone

     The first four days of menstruation and the last four days before menstruation are known as the *paramenstruum*. It is a useful term that is often used in surveys, for these days occur regardless of the length of a woman's cycle. Any adjustment needed due to a cycle being longer or shorter than twenty-eight days is made in the late postmenstruum: in long cycles the postmenstruum will be longer than eight days, while short cycles will have a short postmenstruum.

     Readers should note that the progesterone that is present from ovulation until menstruation is a natural hormone, not to be confused with the synthetic *progestogen* or *progestins* found in the Pill, which have completely different actions (see pages 73–74).

PROGESTERONE LEVELS

Figure 15 shows the relative hormone levels, but since the introduction of radioimmunoassays it has been possible to obtain reliable estimations of hormone levels from a blood sample. Estrogen is present in varying amounts throughout the cycle, being highest at ovulation and again halfway between ovulation and menstruation, and is measured in *picograms*. On the other hand, the blood level of progesterone, which is present only in infinitely small amounts during the first half of the cycle, suddenly rises at ovulation to levels that are measured in *nanograms,* some one thousand times larger than picograms (See Figure 17).

Thus in treatment, the doses of progesterone may need to be some one thousand times greater than estrogen doses. In treatment estrogen is usually given in doses of 0.65 to 1.25 mg daily, so progesterone doses need to be an average of 1,000 mg daily. It must be noted that in the failed clinical trials of progesterone in PMS, the dose of progesterone was always below 1,000 mg, except in the successful PMS double-blind, placebo-controlled trials using 800 mg progesterone by Dr. Pat Magill, reported in the *British Journal of General Practitioners* in 1994 (see page 252).

In pregnancy the placenta produces massive amounts of progesterone, so during pregnancy most PMS sufferers are free from symptoms (Figure 18). During labor the placenta comes away and there is a sudden, drastic fall in the level of progesterone, which too often results in postnatal depression.

Recently, Dr. Kruitwagon and his colleagues in Rotterdam have shown that the level of progesterone in peritoneal fluid is on

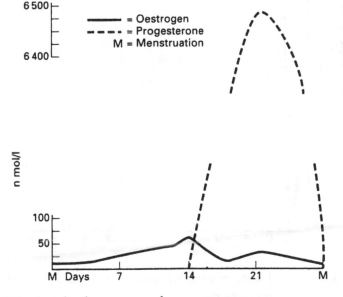

Figure 17   Levels of estrogen and progesterone

PROGESTERONE blood levels are measured
in nanograms.
ESTROGEN blood levels are measured in picograms.
But remember,
PICOGRAMS are one thousand times smaller than
NANOGRAMS.

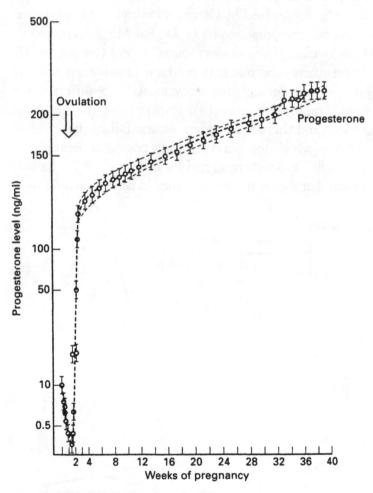

Figure 18   Progesterone levels in the menstrual cycle and pregnancy

average some fifty times higher than the progesterone level in the blood. Unfortunately, whereas it is relatively easy to obtain blood samples for hormone estimations, there are greater difficulties in obtaining peritoneal fluid from within the abdominal cavity.

Progesterone enters the blood in spurts, so to get reliable results one needs to collect several samples on one day and take the average. Moreover, progesterone blood levels decrease following a large meal, which also needs to be considered when interpreting results (see Figure 51). Progesterone blood levels taken seven days before menstruation will demonstrate whether ovulation has occurred that month. A level above 10 ng/ml suggests ovulation has occurred, but one needs to know the date of the test and the date of the first day of the next menstruation.

PROGESTOGENS

Because progesterone cannot be given orally, biochemists tried to make a synthetic preparation that could swallowed. They tried small alterations in the chemical formula, hoping to find a compound with slightly different properties; after all, progesterone, estrogen, testosterone, and cortisone all have very similar formulas, although they have quite different properties. Eventually they developed the *"progestogens,"* or *"progestins,"* which are the basis of all contraceptive pills and gave rise to a multibillion-dollar industry. When the progestogens were first developed, they were believed to be true progesterone substitutes. But, in fact, they had some properties of estrogen, some of progesterone, and some of testosterone. For example, if progestogens have been given during a pregnancy and the child is a girl, she is likely to show masculinizing effects in her genitals and be a tomboy, with marked aggression. This is quite different from the effect of natural progesterone, which is produced in such large quantities during pregnancy. Indeed, surveys have suggested that if progesterone is given to a mother before the sixteenth week of pregnancy for eight weeks or longer, the child of that pregnancy has a tendency toward enhanced intelligence, higher grades, and a better chance of reaching university level than control children whose mothers are not given progesterone (see page 256).

There are many differences between progesterone and the various progestogens, but unfortunately, there are still some doctors who do not realize this. Progesterone lowers the blood pressure, while progestogens raise it; and while progesterone raises the SHBG level, progestogens lower it (see pages 22, 24). Progestogens are not accepted by progesterone receptors. Progesterone can relieve water and sodium retention, whereas some progestogens used in the Pill, such as norethisterone, cause retention of water and sodium. Progesterone is converted by the adrenals into all the various corticosteroids, which is not possible with progestogens. One function of progesterone is to maintain a pregnancy, but the progestogens cannot be used for this purpose. Some progestogens have an estrogenic effect as well, which is useful in the contraceptive field. The disposal of progestogens from the body differs from that of natural progesterone, which is excreted in the urine and feces as pregnanediol.

Progestogens also lower the blood level of progesterone (see Figure 19), and this explains why women with PMS so often have difficulty in tolerating the Pill (see pages 152–154), whether the estrogen-progestogen pill or the progestogen-only pill, and also other estrogen/progestogen preparations for menopause (see page 154).

Some doctors believe that by eliminating ovulation and menstruation with the use of strong progestogens such as danazol, it is possible to eliminate PMS. Unfortunately, this does not happen—it merely prolongs the premenstrual symptoms throughout the cycle. On the other hand, danazol is often the drug of choice in the treatment of endometriosis.

MOLECULAR BIOLOGY

Scientists working with the superpowerful electron microscope have revolutionized medicine and have been able to work out

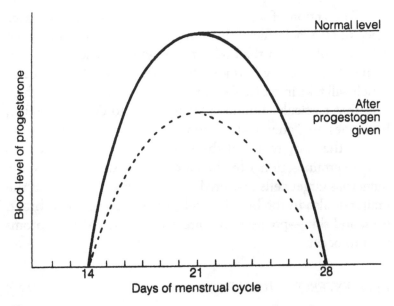

Figure 19   Effect of progestogens on the blood level of
                 progesterone

the actions that occur inside the nuclei of cells. Fifty years ago
students were taught that all the cells in our bodies have a
nucleus, seen as a dark spot when the cells are stained and
observed under a microscope, but we never had any idea of the
importance of this nucleus. Today we have a new branch of science, *nuclear medicine*, and large numbers of molecular biologists are trying to interpret their evidence of what goes on
within the cell nucleus. In the mighty tome *Clinical Gynecologic
Endocrinology and Infertility*, 5th Edition, published in 1994 by
Leon Spiroff, Robert H. Glass, and Nathan G. Kase (Baltimore,
MD: Williams and Wilkins), they write,

> We have entered the age of molecular biology. It won't
> be long before endocrine problems will be explained,
> diagnosed and treated at the molecular level. Soon the
> traditional hormone assays will be a medical practice of
> the past.

The action of a hormone, including progesterone, takes place when a molecule of the hormone reaches the nucleus of a cell. Not all cells in the body are designed to react to all hormones, but for every hormone there are certain "target" cells, which will take in molecules of the hormone and then do whatever that particular hormone "tells" them to do. (Remember, hormones are "chemical messengers," sent by one particular part of the body to signal the target cells in other places to take a certain action.) In the case of progesterone, there are numerous target cells scattered in the body, particularly in the brain but also in the blood vessels, bones, lungs, nose, throat, eyes, and skin—precisely the areas in which PMS symptoms tend to occur.

PROGESTERONE RECEPTORS

Progesterone molecules can pass through a target cell into the cell substance, but on their own they cannot get from there to within the nucleus. Special compounds called progesterone receptors transport progesterone molecules from the cell substance into the cell nucleus, where the progesterone molecule is broken down and does its appointed job. The chemical formula of *progesterone receptors* has been discovered and molecular biologists have already been able to recognize some unique characteristics in these receptors. In 1990 I published my paper "The Aetiology of Premenstrual Syndrome Is with the Progesterone Receptors," the first on that subject, and there has been considerable work on progesterone receptors since. It is now appreciated that those small amounts of progesterone and progesterone receptors are present in both sexes from fetal life until death.

The Cause of Premenstrual Syndrome
Is with the Progesterone Receptors.

The understanding of nuclear biology has ended our reliance on radioimmunoassays in respect to progesterone blood level, which has been found in PMS patients to be normal. A normal progesterone blood level does not mean that there are a normal number of progesterone receptors present in cells, nor does it determine whether the progesterone receptors are functioning well or poorly.

In 1986, Bruce Nock and his colleagues in New York showed that progesterone receptors do not transport progesterone molecules into the nucleus of cells if adrenaline is present. This is most likely to happen in everyday life when we miss a meal and our blood sugar level drops. This explains why the Three-Hourly Starch Diet is advocated (see chapter 24).

It has also been found that progesterone receptors will not transport the artificial progestogens to the nuclei of cells, which explains the failure of artificial progestogens to cure PMS (see page 74), as well as the side effects PMS patients experience with hormonal contraception (see pages 152–154) and estrogen replacement therapy (pages 206–208).

Blaustein and his team working in Amherst, Massachusetts, demonstrated that while the first dose of progesterone can be very small and still act on the nucleus, later doses need to be some forty times higher. In short, after the initial dose of progesterone, the subsequent biochemical reaction in the nucleus becomes less sensitive (hyposensitive) and needs a very high dose of progesterone to stimulate it.

Sites of Progesterone Receptors

Progesterone receptors are found in all vertebrates, including fish, birds, lizards, and snakes, and the recognized laboratory animals such as the guinea pig and mouse. In women the largest concentration of progesterone receptors is in the limbic area of the brain, the area that controls emotions. This is the area animal physiologists call the "area of rage and violence," because if that particular area of the brain is stimulated there is an immediate, violent

---

Unique Characteristics of Progesterone Receptors

They do not transport progesterone
if adrenaline is present.
They do not transport progesterone
if blood sugar levels are low.
They do not transport synthetic progestogens.
They require high doses of progesterone
after the first dose.

---

rage response. This rage response is well known in PMS, with sudden aggression, uncontrolled irritability, and mood swings, and is among the most common of all PMS symptoms. Other areas of the brain also contain progesterone receptors, and scientists have shown that progesterone can act as a monoamine oxidase inhibitor, or MAOI, a type of natural antidepressant (see page 239). Progesterone is also involved in the pathways of dopamine and serotonin, chemicals known to play a part in depression, another common symptom of PMS (see pages 10, 30–31, 34–35, 36–38).

High concentrations of progesterone are also found in cells of the meninges (lining cells of the brain), which are involved in headaches, another common PMS symptom. Other sites where progesterone receptors have been found include the nose, nasal pharyngeal passages, and lungs, accounting for the PMS symptoms of cyclical sore throats, rhinitis, sinusitis, pharyngitis, laryngitis, and asthma. They have been found on the optic pathway in the brain, accounting for the many eye symptoms associated with PMS. The skin, bones, and bladder, as well as the womb, ovaries, and fallopian tubes, all have progesterone receptors, which can cause problems in the premenstruum (see Figure 20).

Breasts contain both estrogen receptors and progesterone receptors, and when cancer is present it is almost invariably due to an excess of estrogen receptors. So while treatment for breast cancer is aimed at reduction of estrogen by medication (tamoxifen is the favorite) or removal of the ovaries, progesterone can still be given.

The specific function of progesterone in the nucleus depends on the particular function of that cell. Thus when progesterone reaches brain cells, it improves the function of brain cells, and when it reaches bone cells, it helps to make new bone cells.

More recently, one particular biological compound, a stress protein called hsp 90, has been isolated inside cells. Molecular biologists think it has the function of regulating the number of progesterone receptors within cells, and work is proceeding to understand the activators and suppressors of progesterone receptors. There is still a considerable amount of work needed before we can fully understand the complete function of progesterone receptors. Unfortunately, there is not yet a suitable test to estimate the number and efficient working of progesterone receptors, which is what doctors treating PMS are waiting for.

PMS Is a Hormonal Disease

- Symptoms are related to the timing of progesterone levels in the premenstruum.
- Symptoms ease during pregnancy when high levels of placental progesterone are present.
- Symptoms recur immediately after pregnancy when there is a sudden loss of placental progesterone.
- Progesterone levels rise a thousand times in the premenstruum.
- Progesterone receptors are needed for the functioning of progesterone.
- The functioning of progesterone is not indicated by measurements of the blood levels of progesterone, which are normal in women with PMS.

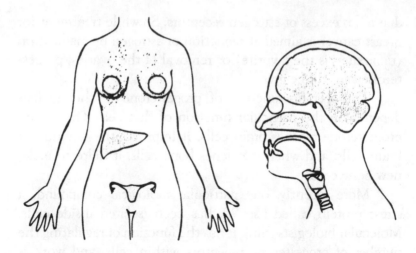

Figure 20   Widespread distribution of progesterone receptors

- Progesterone receptors are present at the sites of PMS symptoms.
- Progesterone receptors do not transport progestogens to the nuclei.
- Progesterone receptors do not function in the presence of adrenaline or low glucose level.
- High doses of progesterone are needed to stimulate progesterone receptors.

7

Ups and Downs of
Progesterone Therapy

Progesterone and PMS are closely linked, although over the decades the strength of these links has varied. Fifty years ago the six initial PMS patients, two of whom suffered from migraines, two from epilepsy, and two from asthma, were all housewives with children. Not only did they all report spontaneously that their symptoms always occurred before menstruation, but it was also noticed that they were well during pregnancy, although they all had severe symptoms immediately after pregnancy.

Characteristics of the First PMS Patients

- Symptoms before menstruation
- Freedom of symptoms during pregnancy
- Severe symptoms immediately after delivery

At that time, the relative levels of the menstrual hormones were as shown in Figure 21, and the level of progesterone during pregnancy in Figure 22.

This suggested that the patients had symptoms in the premenstruum, when their level of progesterone was low, and

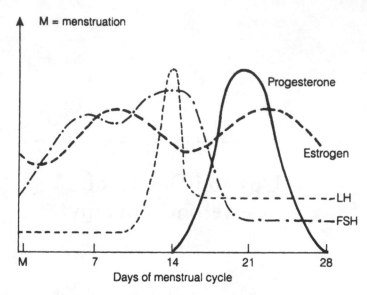

Figure 21 Menstrual hormone variations during the menstrual
cycle

freedom from symptoms during pregnancy, when placenta progesterone gave them sufficient progesterone. Progesterone
treatment was used because progesterone was needed in the
premenstruum when their symptoms were present; placental
progesterone was present in massive amounts during pregnancy, when symptoms were absent; and delivery of the placenta at labor caused a sudden loss of progesterone and severe
symptoms. Progesterone proved to be the right choice and
brought relief to their monthly problems, although progesterone was not much used in those days. Progesterone had
been tried and failed in the treatment of rheumatoid arthritis,
recurrent miscarriages, and severe preeclampsia.

Dr. Raymond Greene and I diagnosed PMS and treated
these patients successfully with progesterone, finally publishing
the results of treatment of eighty-four women with PMS in the
British Medical Journal in May 1953. This was the first-ever publication on PMS that covered all types of premenstrual symptoms, and not just tension. Since those days, our knowledge of

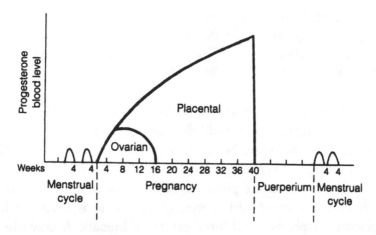

Figure 22 Levels of progesterone during the menstrual cycle and pregnancy

progesterone has grown by leaps and bounds and it is studied in universities throughout the globe. During 1997 alone, over twelve hundred scientific research papers were published in peer-reviewed scientific journals, all discussing different aspects of progesterone, including its action in humans as well as numerous different species of animals. Admittedly, not all the papers were interested in the action of progesterone on women, for breeding and reproduction are also of financial concern to farmers, both on land and in fisheries. While once progesterone was referred to as the "forgotten hormone," it no longer deserves that title in the scientific world, although the new information about progesterone and progesterone receptors is still unknown by the lay public.

Animal Studies Using Progesterone Reported in 1997–1998

Bass	Baboon	Bear	Buffalo	Bush Baby
Cat	Catfish	Chicken	Cow	Deer
Dog	Elephant	Falcon	Frog	Goat
Goldfish	Guinea pig	Hamster	Horse	Lizard

Marmoset	Mink	Monkey	Mouse	Octopus
Pig	Quail	Possum	Rabbit	Rat
Salmon	Sheep	Skate	Talbot	Toad
Turkey	Wallaby	Woodchuck		

It is now recognized that progesterone is the oldest steroid, being some fifty million years old, and is present in all vertebrates, including both sexes of humans, from fetal life until old age. It is readily appreciated that not all vertebrates menstruate nor utilize progesterone for reproduction or menstruation. In lower vertebrates, progesterone is involved in glucose metabolism and intelligence. In humans, it is synthesized in the adrenal glands from amino acids and cholesterol, and the progesterone is then further synthesized and passes into the bloodstream as estrogens, testosterones, and cortisones (stress hormones). In addition, women during their menstruating years make both progesterone and estrogen in their ovaries, while during pregnancy the placenta makes massive amounts of progesterone for the development of the fetus.

During the fifties, progesterone by injection was used for the treatment of PMS and prevention of preeclampsia (high blood pressure and swelling of the ankles). In 1962 my paper "Controlled Trials in the Prophylactic Value of Progesterone in the Treatment of Pre-eclamptic Toxaemia" was published in the *Journal of Obstetrics and Gynaecology of the British Commonwealth* (the name of that journal has since changed to *British Journal of Gynaecology and Obstetrics*). Then came the thalidomide disaster, with the realization that drugs given during pregnancy could affect the unborn child. Reports followed that synthetic progestogens administered in early pregnancy caused masculinization of the female fetus. With the failure of the medical profession to appreciate the difference between natural progesterone and synthetic progestogens (see pages 244–245) the use of progesterone during pregnancy stopped abruptly. As recently as June 1998, Doctors Martorano, Ahlgrimm, and Colbert from PMS Medical Center, New York, described in a medical journal yet again the critical differences between natural progesterone and synthetic progestogens and reminded doctors that synthetic progestogens are not interchangeable with natural progesterone. No further work on the use of progesterone in preventing preeclampsia was undertaken, although progesterone treatment for PMS continued.

During the fifties and sixties surveys were undertaken to emphasize the sociological hazards of the premenstruum in relation to accidents, hospital admissions, behavior, education, and children. Since 1979, English law has accepted PMS in mitigation of crimes, especially murder, arson, and assault, in those cases where the beneficial effect of progesterone had been demonstrated to the court. The women must plead guilty and are then released on probation conditional on continuing supervision of their progesterone treatment for three years (see chapter 19).

The sixties saw the development of progesterone suppositories, which could be inserted rectally or vaginally and used instead of frequent intramuscular injections, needed daily or on alternate days. It was soon established that suppositories needed to be given at least twice daily for any beneficial effect, and that at least two hours were needed between insertions. The maximum effect of each suppository appeared to be 400 mg and lasted for an average of eight to eighteen hours, so the minimum dose of suppositories was 400 mg twice daily, which was the dose later licensed by the British FDA for the treatment of PMS.

PROGESTOGENS IN PREGNANCY

The thalidomide disaster was a worldwide one and brought with it the realization that drugs administered during pregnancy can harm the fetus. It was then shown that progestogens taken during pregnancy could cause masculinization of the female fetus, which is not really surprising, for the synthetic progestogens are derivatives of testosterone (see page 73). Fear entered the medical profession and even natural progesterone, Nature's own pregnancy hormone, was avoided. This meant that my surveys showing increased intelligence in children of mothers given progesterone during pregnancy (see pages 73–74) were ignored, because they could not be confirmed. Perhaps if there is a survey in the near future of the intelligence of in vitro fertilization children, that will open up interest in the subject again, for their mothers would have received progesterone for varying lengths of time during early pregnancy. Also, stopping the use of progesterone brought a halt to its use in preventing the development of preeclampsia in those with symptoms in mid-pregnancy, which has not yet been resumed, although controlled trials reported in 1962 in the *Journal of Obstetrics and Gynaecology of the British Commonwealth* showed the benefit.

In 1980 the first PMS clinic opened in Boston, and it soon had a nationwide clientele. They used the English progesterone suppository, Cyclogest, with success until it was pointed out that Cyclogest was not licensed in the United States, so the import stopped abruptly. Progesterone suppositories were available with a medical prescription, which needed to be taken to a pharmacist, whose task it was to make up the suppositories. The Professional Compounding Company of America (PCCA) in Houston came to the help of pharmacists by supplying them with kits for making up suppositories. There remains a price difference, for in Britain, Cyclogest is available under the National Health Scheme at about half the American price.

PROGESTERONE ESTIMATIONS

Initially, progesterone levels were estimated by measuring the breakdown products of progesterone in a twenty-four-hour collection of urine. This was accepted as an unreliable measurement, because an unknown proportion of the breakdown products was also excreted in the feces. The revolutionary discovery of radioimmunoassays changed the method of measuring the female hormones, because blood samples could be used with greater accuracy. To the surprise of PMS workers, this method showed that low progesterone blood levels were not necessarily associated with PMS. For many doctors who had not personally seen the benefit of progesterone, this was sufficient reason to seek another cause for PMS. At the same time, psychiatrists and psychologists with no experience of hormonal therapy hijacked PMS (see chapter 9), so treatment with psychological methods and psychiatric medication became the norm in America and Australia. The advantage of this was that when the term *LLPDD* (Late Luteal Phase Dysphoric Disorder) was introduced, insurance companies recognized PMS as a disease. But they recognized only the behavioral symptoms of PMS, and not the systemic symptoms such as asthma, migraine, and epilepsy, if these were not accompanied by tension symptoms. Many felt betrayed and disliked a psychological stigma being given to a hormonal disease like PMS.

Radioimmunoassays also revealed the marked differences in the blood levels of estrogen and progesterone, for estrogen is measured in picograms per milliliter, while progesterone is measured in nanograms per liter, which is a thousand times greater, as shown in Figure 17. This means that the relative levels of menstrual hormones shown in Figure 15 do not show the infinitesimal amount of progesterone present in the follicular phase (the time from the end of menstruation until ovulation). It is this infinitesimal amount of progesterone that is present in all humans of both sexes, from the embryo stage until death.

Radioimmunoassays are valuable in determining the absorption of progesterone administered by various methods. Volunteers are tested in their follicular phase, one month with no progesterone and a subsequent month with progesterone either by injection, by vaginal or rectal suppository, orally, or through the skin. These tests have revealed marked differences, with the best absorption being by intramuscular injection, good absorption vaginally and rectally, and poor absorption through the skin and orally.

Free progesterone can also be tested in salivary samples, which are easier for large-scale research studies. In 1994 Dr.

Brian Harris and his team in Cardiff studying postnatal depression reported on 120 volunteers, who were instructed in how to collect samples and asked to collect two samples daily until delivery and then at set times daily for the next thirty-five days. The samples were stored at home in a freezer or refrigerator. The results showed that those who suffered from postnatal blues had a higher progesterone level in late pregnancy and a lower progesterone level after delivery.

IN VITRO FERTILIZATION

For years obstetricians had been trying, but Dr. Steptoe was the first to deliver a child conceived outside the womb. The secret lay in stimulating the inside lining of the womb (endometrium) with progesterone inserted into the vagina, which passed into the womb. This appreciation of the need for progesterone in early pregnancy led to a more general use of progesterone, both in early pregnancy to prevent habitual miscarriages and in the prevention of postnatal depression and PMS. This once again made progesterone therapy medically acceptable, and in 1997 it was estimated that over 50 percent of British GPs used progesterone for PMS.

De Ziegler and colleagues from Paris in 1997 showed that there is a quick passage of progesterone from the vagina to the inner lining of the womb, which makes vaginal administration particularly useful in pregnancy and when progesterone is needed to proliferate the endometrium in certain gynecological diseases.

PROGESTERONE RECEPTORS

Progesterone treatment for PMS was rescued by the molecular biologists using the extreme magnification of the electron microscope to study the chemical reactions within the cells and their nuclei. The molecules of hormones reach the nuclei of their target cells by being transported (or bound) by hormone

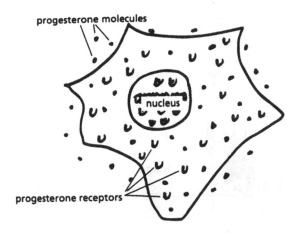

Figure 23   Progesterone molecules and progesterone receptors

receptors, and so progesterone is transported to the nucleus by progesterone receptors. Because progesterone is a steroid, its molecules can move into the cell substance (or cytoplasm) but cannot enter the nucleus without being transported by progesterone receptors. Cells that can metabolize progesterone molecules contain thousands of progesterone receptors (see Figure 23); however, the actual function of the cells by which the progesterone is used varies. Thus, in the brain cells progesterone is involved in behavior, whereas in the bones it is involved in increasing the bone mineral density of individual cells.

Unfortunately, we currently do not have a routine test to estimate the number or effectiveness of the progesterone receptors, although recent work on the by-products of progesterone metabolism within the nucleus, such as allopregnanelone, suggests that the level of these is lower in PMS sufferers. Measuring the levels of such by-products may be the beginning of a new method of diagnosing PMS by a blood test.

The greatest accumulation of progesterone receptors is found in the limbic area of the brain. This is the area of emotion, or the site known by animal physiologists as the "area of rage and violence." The presence of an abnormal level of progesterone receptors here may account for PMS tension, irritability, and

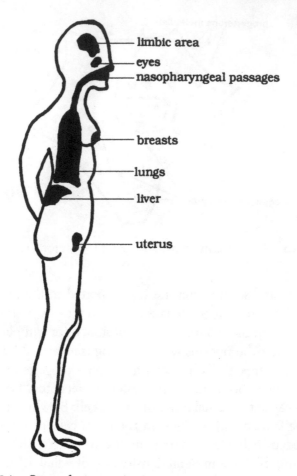

Figure 24   Sites of progesterone receptors

violence. Progesterone receptors are also present in other areas of the brain—the hypothalamus, preoptic area, and meninges—accounting for the frequency of eye symptoms and headaches in PMS sufferers. Progesterone receptors occur in the nasal pharyngeal passages and lungs, accounting for premenstrual rhinitis, sore throats, pharyngitis, laryngitis, and asthma. They are also found in the breasts, liver, bones, fallopian tubes, and skin and hair follicles, all sites of PMS symptoms. The widespread distribution of progesterone receptors in different target cells explains the numerous different symptoms of PMS.

Studies into the characteristics of progesterone receptors have of necessity relied on animal studies, as there have been no normal or PMS volunteers for brain biopsies. Among the known characteristics of progesterone receptors are their inability to bind to artificial progestogens, such as are present in all contraceptive pills, which may explain the difficulty PMS sufferers have in tolerating the Pill.

Dr. Blaustein and his team working in Amherst, Massachusetts, were the first to demonstrate that while the first dose of progesterone can be very small and still act on the nucleus, the second and subsequent doses need to be some forty times higher to stimulate the same action. In short, after the first dose of progesterone, the subsequent chemical action in the nucleus becomes much less sensitive (or hyposensitive) and needs a much higher dose to stimulate it. This must be appreciated when using progesterone in treatment.

Dr. Bruce Nock and his colleagues in New York demonstrated that progesterone receptors do not transport molecules of progesterone to the nucleus in the presence of adrenaline, which occurs at times of stress or if there is a drop in the blood sugar level. This may explain why PMS is always worse at times of extreme stress, something that should be considered in treatment. It is also the reason that PMS treatment should include the Three-Hourly Starch Diet (chapter 24).

There is now sufficient evidence to suggest that the problems of PMS are related to progesterone receptors, but there is still a need for considerably more research to be done on the subject. Research into progesterone receptors is still progressing, and it is now recognized that there are two types of receptors, known as A and B. But their individual functions are not yet understood.

The minutely small progesterone level that is present in both sexes throughout life is now recognized to be essential for the normal cellular functioning of the bones, inner lining cells of the blood vessels (endothelium), myelin covering of nerves, and skin and hair follicles. In the future, scientists will probably discover yet more important uses of progesterone.

8

*

Normal Gynecological Examination

Because the symptoms of PMS are linked to the menstrual cycle, many women first consult a gynecologist hoping that their diagnosis can be confirmed without the need for menstrual recording, but in fact a full gynecological examination will not be able to confirm the diagnosis (see chapter 3). This is because a woman with PMS is likely to have a normal gynecological exam.

At your initial visit to the gynecologist, the first question is likely to be, "When did you have your first menstruation?" This is known as the menarche and is influenced by racial, genetic, dietetic, social, and economic factors. The average age of the menarche in healthy girls in the United States and Britain is 13.1 years, but it varies throughout the world, being highest in the Bundi tribe in New Guinea, at 18.8 years, and lowest in Cuba, at 12.4 years. Among British children attending special schools for the deaf, blind, and physically disabled, the average age is lower, at 12.2 years. It is even lower among those with congenital deformities known to start in early fetal life, such as spina bifida, rubella, and congenital displacement of the hip; for these girls the average age is 10.8 years. On the other hand, the mentally disabled and those with Down's syndrome have a later menarche. Those suffering from a systemic

92

disease such as diabetes or tuberculosis, and especially anorexia, are likely to be late starting menstruation.

Sufferers of PMS tend to have a normal age of menarche. Menstruation is usually quite normal and free from pain, but in retrospect it is remembered as a time of turmoil, crying for no reason, or quarrelling with friends or family. Mothers who suffer from PMS are likely to notice if there are any symptoms, such as sore throat, facial acne, or behavior tantrums, at their daughters' menarche. The first menstruation may last between two and eight days, which may be longer than their mothers expected it to be. There is then usually an interval of between two and six months before the next menstruation occurs unexpectedly. Only about 50 percent of girls have regular menstruation by the age of sixteen.

The most frequent age for women to seek medical help for PMS is in their mid-thirties, but when 1,095 women with PMS were asked retrospectively when their problems first started, 32 percent recalled symptoms during puberty.

Another usual question in a gynecological exam is how often and for how long menstruation now occurs. PMS sufferers tend to have normal menstruation lasting from two to seven days, occurring in cycles from twenty-one to thirty-five days. A cycle length of twenty-eight days is only the average, and very few women, unless they are on the Pill or receiving hormonal medication, have a precise cycle of twenty-eight days for twelve calendar months. At ovulation, the healthy vaginal discharge changes from watery, colorless, and odorless to a thick, opaque, odorless, nonitchy, and stretchy discharge. (If some of the discharge is tested between two sheets of toilet paper, it will stretch.) This is a good sign of normal ovulation and will occur in patients with PMS.

Thus, although patients will be able to describe the horrors of their symptoms that occur each premenstruum, their menstrual history will be normal.

The abdomen will then be examined (or palpated) to ensure that the womb is not enlarged, that the liver and kidneys feel normal and no abnormal masses are detected, and that no free fluid is present. A vaginal speculum will be inserted into the vagina to inspect the vaginal walls and the state of the cervix. A cervical (or Pap) smear will be taken for further examination. Possibly a high vaginal swab will be taken and incubated for a few days to detect any bacterial or thrush infection. In PMS patients, the examination should be normal. If any abnormalities are discovered, they will need to be treated before the PMS.

Blood tests may be taken to determine the levels of progesterone, estrogen, follicle-stimulating hormone (FSH), luteinizing hormone (LH), and prolactin. However, as the levels of these hormones vary over the cycle, it is essential to know accurately the date of the previous menstruation and the expected date of the next menstruation. It is also wise to take a blood test for anemia and general biochemistry. Some may even take a saliva test of progesterone, but as stated earlier, this is irrelevant as it is the progesterone receptors, not the progesterone level, that are at fault in PMS. Again, all these tests are likely to be normal in PMS patients.

A pelvic ultrasound can visualize the size and shape of the womb and ovaries, as well as noting the thickness of the inner lining of the womb (endometrium), which will be shed at menstruation, and show evidence of ovulation and conception. It will exclude the possibility of troublesome fibroids, polyps, and cysts, and it is likely to be normal in PMS patients.

The inside of the womb may be viewed directly with a hysteroscope, an instrument that can be used in the office without an anaesthetic. A minute portion of the lining (biopsy) may be removed for microscopic examination later by a pathologist. This examination has now tended to obviate the need for a D & C (dilatation and curettage) previously so popular, but requiring a general or local anesthetic.

If an abdominal abnormality is suspected, the patient may be advised to have a laparoscopy under a general anaesthetic, with keyhole surgery into the abdominal cavity, allowing the fallopian tubes and ovaries to be seen directly.

All these gynecological examinations would be expected to yield normal results in sufferers of PMS, for as discussed earlier, the menstrual clock does not lie in the womb or ovaries but in the higher central system. The exact site is unknown, but it is possibly in the hypothalamus or adrenals. As discussed in chapter 6, the fault in PMS lies with the progesterone receptors.

This chapter has been written to emphasize the well-recognized fact that if PMS patients do not have any gynecological disease, then the removal of a healthy womb, with or without removal of two healthy ovaries, will be of no benefit to their PMS symptoms, which may even become worse (see chapter 20). There will be relief of monthly bleeding, so they will be discharged from gynecological care, but their premenstrual symptoms will continue.

Nevertheless, PMS is a disease of women, related to their reproductive function, and it should be treated by gynecologists, even if the technology is not yet in place for a simple diagnostic test. Merely trying estrogen and/or progestogen is insufficient; gynecologists should become familiar with progesterone therapy.

9

※

Hijacked by the Psychologists

The Greene and Dalton study in 1953 reported that just 33 percent of PMS sufferers had psychological symptoms, but a different picture emerged when in 1982 another survey in the same English practice was presented to the FDA meeting in Washington to determine the safety of progesterone treatment. Among the 1,095 women receiving progesterone for PMS, there was a preponderance of 55 percent with psychological symptoms. By that time, English law had accepted PMS as a cause of diminished responsibility in cases of murder and serious crimes, and there was general awareness of the psychological symptoms of PMS, which were causing havoc in homes and workplaces.

The first conference convened in 1983 by the National Institute of Mental Health established diagnostic guidelines for PMS and affirmed the interest of mental health professionals in women suffering from premenstrual mood swings. In 1987, PMS was defined as the Late Luteal Phase Dysphoric Disorder (LLPDD), which was included as a proposed clinical diagnosis in an appendix of the *Diagnostic and Statistical Manual of Mental Disorders*. This meant that PMS was accepted as a disease for insurance purposes, and while many people were upset by it being considered a psychological rather than hormonal disease, the advantages outweighed the psychological stigma. In 1994, the terminology changed, and PMS was classified as Premenstrual Dysphoric Disorder and placed under the section "Depression not Otherwise Specified." The definition covers an increase in premenstrual symptoms, with a diminution of symptoms in the follicular phase; thus it may cover menstrual magnification. So the takeover by psychologists occurred with no objection from the medical profession, for there is no one specialty dealing with PMS.

In 1982 I was given a VIP tour of the National Institutes of Health in Bethesda. It started in the entrance hall, where there was a model of the building on a central table. The helpful official showed me the areas where research and work was proceeding in the various specialties. His finger pointed in turn to the many departments dealing with the heart, lungs, brain, stomach, eyes, kidney, liver, and so on. To my question of where was the work on PMS proceeding, he answered briefly, "In the cracks." That expressed exactly what appears to have happened in America, a country that is leading the field in so many other branches of medicine.

In England, 95 percent of the population is registered under the National Health Service with a general practitioner, who keeps the medical records and passes them on to the next doctor whenever patients move. Most general practitioners there see the whole patient, with either physical or psychological symptoms, and are good at recognizing PMS, for which 65 percent prescribe progesterone. Furthermore, among the categories of patients entitled to free prescriptions are those on social security and patients with endocrine disorders; the others pay a nominal sum for any progesterone. PMS may be accepted by the English courts as mitigation for an offense (see pages 172–173). This means general practitioners may be asked by the court for a report, or possibly to produce medical records. So they tend to record the presence or absence of PMS or the date of the last menstruation, if that is considered important.

The problem with psychologists is that many of them have had no medical background, few have examined naked women, inserted a speculum in the vagina, used an auroscope to view an inflamed ear drum, or placed a stethoscope on the chest to hear the high-pitched squeak of asthma. Furthermore, their knowledge of hormones probably ended when they were in college and has not been updated since. Few appreciate the different measures used for estrogen and progesterone blood levels, the latter of which is one thousand times greater than the former (see pages 70–73, 87).

I became aware of this abysmal lack of background medicine when a psychiatric consultant asked me to see Toni.

Toni had been admitted the previous month, settled down well, but then had another psychotic attack while in hospital. She was twenty-five, and I had known her since she was an attractive, petite teenager. She had PMS and could not tolerate the pill, so she had twice needed to terminate a pregnancy, and on both occasions her PMS had increased in severity. She was not very regular with progesterone therapy, forgetting it when she felt well. I was met at the large, south London mental hospital by the consultant, who gave me a brief account of her behavior, introduced me to Toni, and asked me to go to the nursing office at the end of the consultation. Toni handed me her menstrual chart, and the problem was obvious. She had been admitted for being rowdy and undressing in the shopping mall. She couldn't remember much about it, but knew she had been admitted yet again to the hospital just before menstruation. Within a day or two she had recovered and was allowed to attend occupational therapy, doing pottery that she enjoyed. They would not allow her to restart progesterone, with the result that she had again become confused and rowdy three days before I met with her; she had started menstruating the day before my visit.

When I reported to the consultant, the staff was just having their evening meeting, and I joined in. Seated around the room were the senior and junior registrars, a student, a psychologist, a social worker, a nursing officer, and a staff nurse. I gave my brief account, explaining that Toni's outburst on Friday had been followed on Sunday by her normal menstruation. The nursing staff disagreed, saying she had menstruated ten days earlier. One after another they supported each other, although there was no mention of menstruation in her notes. I had known Toni well enough and relied on her menstrual chart, but it was something that could easily be solved by taking a vaginal swab. I asked the nursing officer if she could arrange it, and she asked for a volunteer. There were no offers, so I agreed to take a swab; within a few minutes I was able to produce a bloodstained swab, which settled the matter. Toni was allowed to restart progesterone treatment and was discharged.

There is at least one psychiatric hospital in southern England where menstrual charts are used and are completed for all women between fifteen and fifty years. It has resulted in changes in the treatment of several patients.

Psychologists and psychiatrists do recognize other hormonal disorders that have psychological and physical symptoms, such as thyroid excess, which causes anxiety; thyroid deficiency, which causes depression and exhaustion; and hypoglycemia, which can lead to aggression and irritability. However, most psychologists and psychiatrists do not even recognize the differences between premenstrual depression and a depressive illness, and will tend to treat both with antidepressants or psychotherapy. Depression, which can occur in men or women, may last weeks, months, or years, but PMS depression lasts only fourteen days, and by definition there is always a spell of normality between the attacks. Individuals who are depressed tend to lose their appetite and lose weight, but PMS sufferers tend to have food cravings and gain weight. Depressed individuals tend to have sleeping problems, often waking early in the morning, when they wander about the house, maybe make a cup of tea, or even do some housework. PMS sufferers yearn for sleep; they would prefer to stay in bed till midday or longer. There is a decrease in libido in the depressed, but in PMS sufferers there tends to be an increased sex interest, sometimes even an excessive sexual urge. The underlying pathology is different, PMS being a hormonal disease.

Among the reasons given by psychologists and psychiatrists for not considering PMS a hormonal disease is that PMS is not universally relieved by a single treatment—but neither is diabetes, which is a hormonal disease. Menstrual cycles are disturbed by stress, but then, so are numerous other disorders, both physical and psychological. PMS has a genetic factor, noticed in twins and adopted daughters, but so have many other hormonal disorders.

Psychologists rely on two factors in not classifying PMS as a hormonal disorder. One is that the progesterone blood level is within normal levels in women with PMS. However, as I have mentioned, molecular biologists have shown that it is not the progesterone blood level that is involved in PMS but the functioning of progesterone receptors. The other factor is the failure to respond to low-dose progesterone in double-blind placebo-controlled trials, although Dr. P. Magill's multicentered trial of PMS patients using 400 mg twice daily, reported in the *British Journal of General Practitioners* in 1994, showed benefit. No consideration is given to the normal rise in hormone blood levels in which estrogen is measured in picograms and progesterone in nanograms, some one thousand times higher.

Although psychologists need to consider PMS a hormonal disorder responding to progesterone therapy, the sociological effects are within their specialty and are discussed in chapters 10 and 19, dealing with education and legal aspects.

10

—— ?● ——

Education and PMS

The effect of PMS is already evident in the premenarcheal schoolgirl. What does that mean during college life? Premenstrual memory loss and difficulty with recall may still occur later and is noticed by sufferers and their employers, but premenstrual memory loss and difficulty with concentration are not so easily studied in the workplace. The almost universal use of the Pill today is hampering research into the effects of PMS on schoolgirls, but my first studies, reported in my papers "Effect of Menstruation on Schoolgirls' Weekly Work" and "Schoolgirls' Behaviour and Menstruation," both published in the *British Medical Journal* in 1960, were done before young girls used hormonal contraception.

SCHOOLGIRLS' WEEKLY WORK

I studied the effects of menstruation on girls at a top boarding school, where there would not be so much day-to-day influence of home affairs. The girls were required to sign a book when they collected sanitary protection during menstruation. The study covered 1,560 weekly grades in seven to twelve different subjects. Each grade was compared with that of the previous week, and it was noticed that the standard of work fell

101

below the norm by 10 percent during the premenstrual week in comparison with a rise of 20 percent during the postmenstrual week. Furthermore, this pattern of premenstrual fall and postmenstrual rise was equally present in all age groups; it occurred in girls with only one menstruation a term and those who were menstruating each month; it was equally distributed among the bright girls and the duller ones, and among the consistent and the inconsistent girls (Figure 25).

With so much work today involved in school projects, it is worth remembering to complete these, if possible, during the

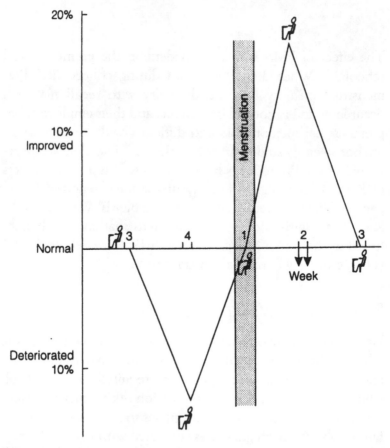

Figure 25   Variations in schoolgirls' weekly grades with menstruation

postmenstrual week, albeit early, rather than in the premenstrual week, when reduced concentration and mental ability may preclude a high grade. In later life this is a useful point to remember if your work depends on deadlines.

EXAMINATIONS

In 1968 my paper "Menstruation and Examinations" was published in *The Lancet*. It studied girls at the same boarding school, those taking the ordinary "O" level public examinations at the average age of sixteen, and those taking the advanced "A" level examination at the average age of eighteen. It showed that those girls who were unfortunate enough to take their examination in the paramenstruum (four days before and the first four days of menstruation) had fewer passes, lower grades, and fewer distinctions. It also appeared that among the ninety-one "O" level candidates it was the girls whose menstruation lasted six or more days who had most failures (Figure 26).

In addition, the girls with long cycles of thirty-one days or more had more failures than did girls with shorter cycles (Figure 27).

Stress of Examinations

Stress is a factor that can alter the timing of menstruation and increase PMS. The effect of stress on the ninety-one schoolgirls taking "O" level public examinations illustrated this. Whereas an average of sixteen girls were menstruating on any one day during the month of May, during examination week in June as many as thirty-six girls were menstruating on one day (Figure 28).

BEHAVIOR

In the same boarding school, it proved possible to analyze the punishments the schoolgirls had received in relation to their menstruation. A total of 272 offenses had been committed

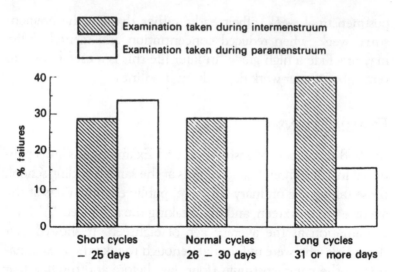

Figure 26   "O" level failures and duration of menstruation

during the fourteen days before and the fourteen days after the first day of menstruation. It was found that the statistically significant figure of 29 percent of all offenses had been committed during the first four days of menstruation, which compares with an expected incidence of 14 percent had there been an even distribution (Figure 29).

Even more interesting was the finding about the sixth-form prefects, aged sixteen to eighteen, who were allowed to punish other girls for misbehavior. They gave significantly more punishments during their own menstruation. Their standards tended to rise with each menstruation and then gradually fall in the postmenstruum (Figure 30). The same is true of teachers, and many a sixth-form girl will watch the day-to-day irritability or calmness of her teacher to decide when it is a good moment to hand in an essay or ask a favor.

TIDINESS

The effect of menstruation on tidiness was demonstrated in the dormitory of another London school, where every morning the

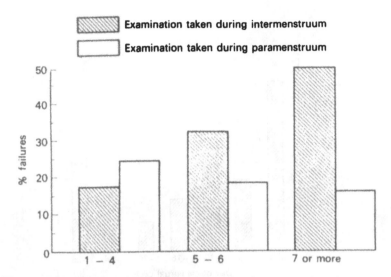

Figure 27   "O" level failures and length of menstrual cycle

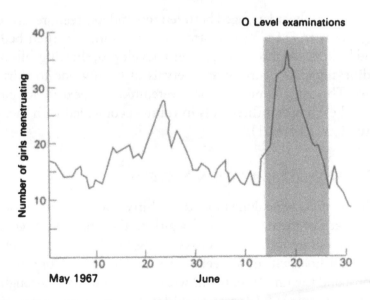

Figure 28   Time of menstruation of ninety-one examination
candidates

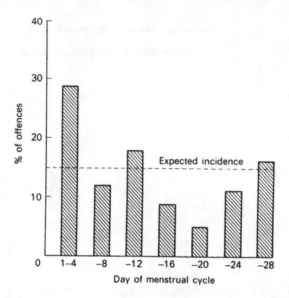

Figure 29   Schoolgirls' punishments during the menstrual cycle

twenty-four boarders, aged between ten and fourteen, received a grade A to D from the matron for the tidiness of their beds and lockers. An interesting pattern developed, showing falls in tidiness grades occurring at intervals of twenty-one to thirty days. The dates of menstruation were unknown, except for girl 1, and each of her three falls in tidiness coincided with menstruation (Figure 31).

CHANGED EXAMINATION SYSTEMS

Those studies were done more than thirty years ago, and notice was taken of them, so that today girls in England have as good a chance at examinations as boys. In the old days examinations were all held within a week, with several compulsory questions, and the unfortunate girl who had worked hard throughout the previous two years could fail just because the examination was on the wrong day of the month. Two years wasted and try again in another year. There was no appeal, certainly not for the unspeakable complaint of PMS. Over time, more

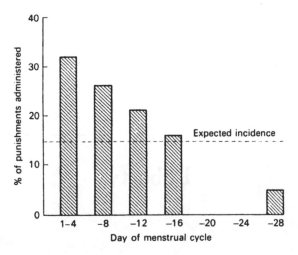

Figure 30   Punishments administered by prefects during their menstrual cycle

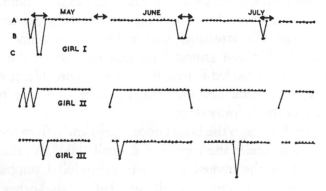

Figure 31   Daily tidiness grades with cyclical drops

emphasis was placed on projects and work done throughout the year, which are now taken into consideration. In British public examinations, if there are two papers on the same subject they must be spaced at least eight days apart, so that the girl cannot be in her paramenstruum for both papers. The teacher's opinion is considered, and appeals are permitted. This consideration has spread to many countries besides Britain and removes some of the menstrual handicap.

11

~~~ ❧ ~~~

Puberty

The menarche, or first menstruation, is an important milestone in any girl's life and demonstrates that she has an intact hormonal pathway from the hypothalamus to the womb. It is heralded over a period of about two years by the appearance of secondary sex characteristics, such as breast development, the growth of pubic and armpit hair, and changes of the body shape into the rounded female figure (see Figure 32). It is not the end of pubertal development, however, and only represents about the halfway stage.

The changes in the breast occur very slowly, from the first development under the nipple of a small "bud" the size of a grape, through the gradual increase in size to full development. Often one breast develops slightly before the other, but although this inequality usually causes much worry and immediate medical advice is sought, there is no cause for alarm. In due course, both breasts will develop equally, for the growth stimulus comes from hormones in the bloodstream.

The attitude taken toward pubertal development depends very much on the culture and society to which a girl belongs. In India and Sri Lanka the first menstruation is a cause for celebration, as it represents a girl's attainment of physical maturity and the beginning of her sexual and reproductive life. The

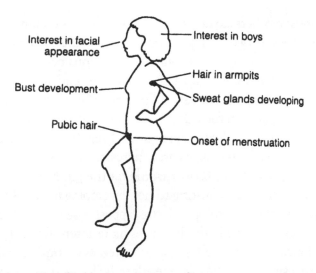

Interest in facial appearance

Bust development

Pubic hair

Interest in boys

Hair in armpits

Sweat glands developing

Onset of menstruation

Figure 32 Female development at puberty

occasion is marked by a change from wearing short dresses to dressing in colorful and beautiful saris. In Pakistan it is reported that the girls in some households are deliberately fed a low-protein diet in order to delay menarche, thus postponing the cost of the marriage, which is expected to occur immediately after the menarche has taken place.

In societies such as Japan and Hong Kong, where the subject was taboo until quite recently, girls obtained information about their changes furtively, from the pages of popular magazines. In the United States, on the other hand, the media forces sex education on every occasion, and it is discussed so freely at home and school that the menarche is almost a nonevent, of more interest to the mother than the girl. In any culture, however, the only girl in a male-dominated family may fear the menarche because it emphasizes the differences between her and her brothers, and it may increase the conflict over her developing femininity.

The first menstruation usually lasts between three and eight days, with an average of five days, which is rather longer than most mothers expect it to be. Then there is usually an interval of between two and six months before the next menstruation. Typically, only about four menstruations occur during the first year after menarche, with the cycle gradually becoming shorter. By the age of sixteen, 20 percent of girls still have cycles that last longer than forty days, and 33 percent have a prolonged bleeding lasting at least seven days. Irregular menstruation is quite common for teenagers and there are many normal reasons for this, though it can be worrisome for the girl herself. In these years she is not only adjusting to her developing figure, she is also becoming more conscious of the opposite sex. As boyfriends come into the picture, she becomes more interested in her own appearance and, all in all, these are often emotion-laden days.

In a single girl the cycle tends to be long—perhaps thirty-five days—but as she begins to be stimulated by contact with boyfriends, her cycle may shorten by a few days and approach the conventional norm, for the menstrual hormones are stimulated by male contact. However, if the male contact is broken and she returns to female companionship, her cycle usually returns to its original pattern.

One nineteen-year-old inquired,

My periods were always very irregular, with sometimes even eight weeks between them. When I first met John they became better, once as short as twenty-eight days. Then we had an awful fight and I broke up with him. Since then, my cycles only seem to come when they want to, every five or six weeks. Does it matter?

At nineteen years of age it does not matter, and probably even before she received a reply she would have found another boyfriend and her menstruation would have become more regular again.

Ovulation first occurs about two years after menarche, not necessarily every month, initially, but every two or three months. Gradually, the cycles become more regular. It is with the onset of ovulation that spasmodic dysmenorrhea might begin. This usually comes as a surprise to both the girl and her mother, as previously menstruation had been so pain-free.

If the spasmodic dysmenorrhea is bad enough to require regular medication for the relief of pain, especially if the girl has to take time off school or work or stay in bed, then medical help should be sought. Years ago it was interesting to listen to mothers explain why they did not take their daughters to the doctor when the girls were suffering from spasmodic dysmenorrhea:

I don't want to be considered fussy or neurotic.

He'll only tell her to get married and have children like I was told!

I would hate for her to have an operation.

He might put her on the Pill and she's too young for that—besides she doesn't have any boyfriends yet.

Boys would take advantage of her if she were on the Pill.

Today it has all changed: the Pill is freely available, and some girls start taking it early, ostensibly to ensure regular menstruation. No more D & Cs (dilatation and curettage) or stretching the opening of the womb under an anesthetic, which used to be the standard treatment for painful periods, or indeed any gynecological problem. Now hormones can do the trick and ease spasmodic dysmenorrhea. If the parents really object to the Pill, the doctor can always prescribe just estrogen, which is not a contraceptive by itself but will ease her monthly pains. Moreover, since the introduction of prostaglandin inhibitors, estrogen and the Pill are no longer the only effective treatments available.

Even before the first menstruation, cyclical mood swings may occur, and they may continue at times of missed menstruation (see Figure 4). These mood swings can transform a happy schoolgirl into a lazy, bad-tempered, selfish grouch whose academic work and behavior deteriorate even before menstruation is established (see *Jessica*, pages 256–257). As a pattern it is very suggestive of PMS, and the mood swings should be recorded so that help can be given to the girl before she falls too far behind in school.

A survey in 1983 of 1,095 patients whom I had treated with progesterone therapy for PMS during the previous thirty years revealed that 57 percent of the 326 childless women had started experiencing PMS at puberty. Most reported that after a few obnoxious years their PMS eased, but then it returned following a successful pregnancy or after some years on the Pill. This emphasizes the importance of considering the possibility of PMS in cases where the teenager is behaving badly, has unexpected mood swings, or becomes a changed person. An additional problem with teenagers is that menstruation is usually irregular for the first few years, so the connection of their odd behavior with menstruation is not so easily made.

In a study of eighteen women with PMS who had a criminal record and were still under twenty-five, it was found that their first episode of unusual behavior had been noticed within six months of their first menstruation. But on the average it was some five years later that the diagnosis of PMS was made and treatment started.

These years may be marked by conflicts between the early maturers and those who mature more slowly. Long-term friendships may break up as one girl develops sooner than another. With maturation comes an interest in boys and a concern about appearance, so that girls spend hours caring for their face and body. At this time, grease starts developing in the skin and the sweat glands begin to operate, so that skin care and deodorants become necessary.

Many girls do not like the body changes that Nature has decreed. They object to the rounded contours and would prefer the broad shoulders and wiry limbs of boys. This stimulates the urge to diet, even in those who are not particularly overweight. Excessive dieting during these developing years is dangerous. It may halt menstruation and ovulation, and lead to anorexia nervosa, with weight loss accompanied by food phobias, and psychological changes. It is not unusual to find girls who reduce their weight from 120 pounds to 70 pounds within a few months by strict dieting and still complain about their body and imagine that they are too fat. Unhappily, the road to recovery in such cases is slow and, if they develop multicystic ovaries, their future fertility is at stake. More recently it has been appreciated that those who have had anorexia are likely at the menopause to be at increased risk of developing osteoporosis, or brittle bone disease. When menstruation does return, it is often accompanied by unpleasant premenstrual symptoms.

Unfortunately for many teenagers, these sexual developments may occur at just the same time as their mothers are experiencing the difficult years of menopause and are also subject to mood swings and unpleasant symptoms. It is important to help adolescents through this stage, however, no matter how impossible and thoughtless they become. They need every opportunity to mix freely with older girls and women, and also with boys and men, to help them sort themselves out and appreciate the differences in individuals, both in men and in women.

Another concern is the increased sex drive that may occur premenstrually. This often causes problems for young adolescents, who may be quite unprepared for this new sex urge and may be unable to control their emotions. The increased sex drive may be responsible for young girls running away from home or custody, only to be found following boys in clubs and at school. These girls can be helped, and their problem behavior frequently disappears if they receive appropriate treatment.

In puberty, premenstrual depression is usually worse than the tiredness and is likely to make a girl sulky, secretive, withdrawn, and anxious to be alone. A careful watch should be kept on her behavior. Too often, the mood swings will occur suddenly, without warning or provocation, and she may make an unexpected suicide attempt.

Phyllis, seventeen years old, had been at the top of her class when she was twelve, and her work had been the envy of others. Gradually, however, she went downhill in both work and behavior. She became sloppy, rude, and bored with everything, gave up any attempt at graduating from high school, and dropped out of school at the first opportunity. She first worked in a hairdressers' salon, but her work was unsatisfactory and her timekeeping poor. Her next job was as a filing clerk, where she felt unappreciated. There would be days when she would come home, slip up to her bedroom, and stay there for hours, allowing no one to enter and refusing food. One day her father found her in a corner, apparently asleep. The doctor diagnosed an overdose of hypnotics and she had to be rushed to the hospital. This incident shocked her mother, who then started to keep a careful eye on her daughter. Soon she noted the correlation between Phyllis's mood swings and menstruation, and she asked for medical help. With treatment her daughter improved quickly, restarted her social life, which had been absent for five years, and later returned to night school.

Teenage girls with PMS should get proper treatment. Initially this means full instruction in the Three-Hourly Starch Diet (see chapter 24), and only if this is strictly adhered to without satisfactory results should progesterone treatment also be necessary. Progesterone treatment is usually only temporary; as the girls mature the need for regular medication decreases, although they may need it again in times of stress. There are a few schools in England that appreciate the need for teenage girls to eat little and often, and they time the school breaks to encourage children to divide up their day's food into the Three-Hourly Starch Diet.

The next chapter is written by my granddaughter, describing in her own words what the pubertal years were like for her.

12

PMS in Adolescence

Jennie Holton

As the granddaughter of a PMS specialist and the daughter of the founding member of PMS Help, suffering from PMS should have been the last thing you expected me to be. However, there is a saying about doctors' families being ignored, and that certainly was the case with me. The problem with diagnosing PMS in adolescents is that teenagers are expected to be moody, uncooperative, antisocial, aggressive, and generally unpleasant, so any behavior that may be correlated with PMS is often just put down to teen angst.

Puberty is a tough time for any girl. I was lucky in that it was discussed quite openly in my family, and I knew the mechanics of what was happening. However, I don't think that any teenager is fully prepared. It's frightening when your body starts changing—your breasts grow, facial spots start appearing, and your body starts filling out. We never really discussed it among friends, apart from guessing who had started their periods and who hadn't, but I'm sure that everyone was feeling just as uncomfortable in their new body as I was.

My periods started when I was thirteen, and almost immediately my problems began. My first symptoms were the typical irritability, mood swings, and tearfulness: I would cry over the slightest thing and was convinced that everyone hated me. Teenage girls can be unpleasant at the best of times, but I would take even the slightest comment toward me the wrong way, and I would end up in the restroom at school crying for quite literally hours at a time. At my worst, I locked myself in the school restroom for about an hour and was almost hysterical by the time one of the teachers managed to coax me out. However, even this event didn't alert anyone to the problem; once again, it was all put down to adolescence.

My relationship with my family deteriorated to the point that I could barely hold a civil conversation with my mother. Often there is the added difficulty that the mother of the adolescent sufferer is going through the menopause, with its related problems. These women are also subject to mood swings and other unpleasantness. Siblings may be caught up in the PMS—with resentment if they don't also suffer from it, or huge arguments if they do. Things are made especially bad by the fact that females who live in close proximity often menstruate at the same time. It certainly held true for our household.

During the next few years my behavior and problems worsened. I became very, very depressed and too lethargic to leave the house. I would become violent toward my sister; because we had a working mother, we were both in the house on our own in the early evenings, and I would take all my frustration out on her. My binge eating was getting out of control; within minutes of getting to school I would have eaten my packed lunch, and then I would go to the candy store four or five times during the rest of the day. At my all-girls school, eating problems were de rigueur, and girls going to lunch to actually eat were seen as greedy and weak. My constant bouts of eating didn't go unnoticed, nor did the fact that I was slightly overweight, although I was never really teased or bullied about it. I was certainly aware of it. I would come home from school, and eat solidly: cakes, pastries, biscuits, sweets—in fact, anything I could get my hands on—and would blame it all on my

sister. Then I would eat a full meal with my family and go to
bed depressed about how fat and ugly I was. My self-esteem
plummeted, and I had no social life at all. Far from being the
best days of my life, school was hell.

Various studies have stated that teenagers aren't more
prone to PMS than older women; however, the results can be
just as devastating. Over the two years that I suffered badly I
missed countless hours of school. Either I wouldn't go at all, or
I would go but end up in the bathroom or hiding on the play-
ground. Sufferers may find their concentration span short-
ened, and simple tasks become impossible as lethargy sets in.
Research in a girls' boarding school by Dr. Dalton, back in the
1960s, showed that grades went down before menstruation but
rose after (see Figure 25). This can cause problems in exams—
if they fall at the wrong time, then results may be poorer, with
more failures and less distinctions—although the advent of
project-based courses in England will put all girls on an equal
footing. Similarly, records of the punishments received by girls
proved that they were more likely to be punished during the
premenstruum than after (see chapter 10). Upon further
investigation, it was even discovered that there is a relationship between the punishments given out by the older girls and
their own menstrual cycles. This obviously raises important
questions about any women in authority—magistrates, police-
women, lawyers, and so on.

It is important that schoolgirl sufferers organize their
work as much as possible so that their workload is lighter in
the premenstruum. General good study techniques should be
learned: working at a set time, in a set place, with no distrac-
tions like TV or telephones (soft music excepted; I myself
work better with a CD on). Taking frequent breaks is one way
of combating a wandering mind, as is switching tasks.

I think that all parents, teachers, social workers, and anyone in contact with adolescent girls should be aware that they
are just as likely to suffer from PMS as women in any other age
group. My PMS was finally recognized when my mother started

making a note of my symptoms, together with the dates of my periods. After only a few months it became clear that I was not acting like as monster all of the time, and that for two weeks a month my behavior was acceptable. She sat me down and discussed it with me, and I immediately started on the Three-Hourly Starch Diet. At first I refused to stick to it strictly—try telling any teenage girl that she is going to have to eat regularly, especially when the recommended foods are potato- and flour-based. However, once I realized that I was not going to have to eat more, but instead to divide up my meals, I decided to give it a try. My mother's most persuasive argument was that at least it should stop my bingeing, which it did. In fact, within a few weeks I no longer had the wild mood swings and was able to concentrate on my lessons for the first time in ages.

Many, many PMS sufferers forget the good times in the two weeks after their period and instead remember only the bad times. I became convinced that I was just a "bad" person. I felt that just as some people are happy, some are sad, and that was just my lot in life—I was a "nasty" person. It did not matter that I had plenty of friends, who ignorèd my bizarre behavior, a loving family, and a great time for half the month—I forgot about that. In fact, if anything, it made me even more depressed to think that I was putting the people I loved through all that. Please don't think that apart from the PMS I was a little angel. I certainly wasn't that, and after the diagnosis and treatment I still had odd bouts of unacceptable behavior, just like any teenage girl. However, I certainly was not really the monster that I behaved like, and I think it is vital that those in contact with teenage girls be aware that PMS may be the cause of some of their extreme behavior.

13

❧

Pain and Periods

A very welcome and much-needed breeze of common sense wafted through the medical and gynecological fields when Doctors Jean and John Lennane, a husband-and-wife team, pointed out in a well-reasoned paper on a group of disorders including period pain that there is no justification for the old idea that "it is all in the mind." Indeed, all existing scientific evidence points toward a hormonal imbalance being the cause of PMS. The Lennanes cite a number of examples from current medical textbooks, which they suggest have led to an irrational and ineffective approach to the treatment of such disorders. These examples included the following:

> It is generally acknowledged that this condition is much more frequent in the "highly strung," nervous, or neurotic female than in her more stable sister.

> Faulty outlook . . . leading to an exaggeration of minor discomfort . . . may even be an excuse for not doing something that is disliked.

> The pain is always secondary to an emotional problem.

119

Very little can be done for a patient who prefers to use menstrual symptoms as a monthly refuge from responsibility and effort.

The idea that period pain, or dysmenorrhea, is purely psychological became widely accepted because there are no abnormalities that can be detected by a physical or gynecological examination, nor are there any suitable tests of hormone levels that can distinguish those who suffer once a month. However, it is gradually being accepted that dysmenorrhea is caused by an imbalance of hormones.

There are two quite different, and in fact opposite, types of dysmenorrhea. One is not PMS; the other is. They are rarely differentiated by the general public, but their treatment is quite different, so it is essential to distinguish between them. There is *spasmodic dysmenorrhea*, characterized by spasms of abdominal pain, which is not PMS, because there is an absence of symptoms in the premenstruum. The other type is *congestive dysmenorrhea* (or PMS), in which there is increasing congestion, pain, and other symptoms during the premenstruum. Congestive dysmenorrhea has all the characteristics of PMS, in addition to period pain, and so is really PMS. The differences between the two types are clearly shown in the table that follows later in this chapter.

SPASMODIC DYSMENORRHEA

When menstruation first starts, at puberty, there is no ovulation, nor is there any period pain. About two years later, however, ovulation commences, and quite unexpectedly, spasmodic dysmenorrhea may begin. Often, at the beginning, ovulation does not occur every month but only in alternate months, so period pain occurs only in alternate months. Spasmodic dysmenorrhea is most frequent between the ages of fifteen and twenty-five. It ends abruptly after a full-term pregnancy, or it may end gradually, with each period becoming less painful during the early twenties. The woman usually feels very well during the premenstruum and then is suddenly doubled up with severe spasms of pain in the lower abdomen on the first day of menstruation. The pains are colicky in nature, coming about every twenty minutes and lasting about five minutes; in fact, they are similar to true labor pains. The girl obtains most relief curling up around a hot water bottle, and aspirin or paracetamol or antiprostaglandin may help take the edge off the pain. The pain may become so severe that bed is the only refuge, and it may continue throughout the night, preventing sleep. A monthly absence from school or work is often necessary.

The pain is easier on the second day and is gone by the third or fourth day. The distribution of pain is in the "bikini" area, as shown in Figure 33; in fact, it covers the area served by the uterine and ovarian nerves. The severity of the pain continues relentlessly on the first day of menstruation, month after month, and is not affected by stress. It is eased by using the Pill, which stops ovulation, and it may be helped, temporarily at least, by an operation popularly known as a D & C (dilatation and curettage), used to stretch the opening of the womb. The girl experiencing dysmenorrhea is often undeveloped, with sparse hair in her armpits and lower abdomen, small breasts with pink nipples, and acne.

It seems that spasmodic dysmenorrhea is caused by there being insufficient estrogen for maturing and stretching the muscles of the womb. During pregnancy there is an abundance of estrogen from the placenta for a full nine months, and the muscle wall of the womb is stretched by the fetus. As a result, this type of period pain usually ends after pregnancy, and it is rare for the woman to subsequently suffer from PMS.

Sufferers of spasmodic dysmenorrhea are often advised to exercise more or to relax more. As part of a survey for the British consumer magazine *Which?* some years ago, more than two hundred women with spasmodic dysmenorrhea kept a careful record of the pain they suffered for at least three cycles. As it

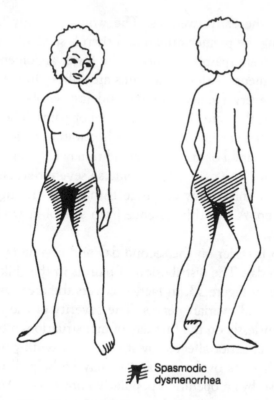

Spasmodic
dysmenorrhea

Figure 33   Site of pain in spasmodic dysmenorrhea

happened, the survey took place in the summer when many were on vacation. The women who normally had active jobs, like waitresses or nurses, tended to choose restful vacations lying in the sun. The others who had more sedentary occupations chose active holidays, cycling five hundred miles, mountaineering, and surfing. Regardless of their usual occupations or level of exercise, however, the amount of pain they experienced was not affected by the exercise or relaxation they had while on vacation.

When cells are damaged, a chemical called prostaglandin is released. In women with spasmodic dysmenorrhea, a high level of prostaglandin F-2-alpha is secreted by the cells of the lining of the womb. Certain drugs known as *prostaglandin inhibitors* are most effective in relieving this type of pain.

Differences Between Spasmodic and Congestive PMS Dysmenorrhea

	Spasmodic	*Congestive*
Start of pain	First day of period	Up to 14 days before period
Site of pain	Lower abdomen, back, inner thighs	Lower abdomen, back, head, breasts, joints, and limbs
Type of pain	Comes in spasms	Heavy, dragging, and continuous, increasing as menstruation starts
Time of starting	2 years after menarche	Before menarche, after the Pill, or at pregnancy
Usual age	15–25 years	13–53 years
Ovulation	Must be present	May be present or absent
Premenstrual symptoms	Absent	Present
Effect of stress	Unrelated	Increases symptoms
After pregnancy	Cured	Increased symptoms
Effect of pill	Cures	Increases symptoms
Treatment	Prostaglandin inhibitors, estrogen, or the pill	Progesterone and a 3-hourly starchy diet

CONGESTIVE DYSMENORRHEA

Congestive dysmenorrhea is the presence of heavy, continuous lower abdominal pain during the last seven days of the premenstruum. The pain increases in severity on the first day of menstruation and then gradually eases, together with the end of the other premenstrual symptoms. In contrast to spasmodic dysmenorrhea, sufferers of congestive dysmenorrhea may experience pain at their first menstruation and continue with it throughout their menstrual life, and the symptoms are present whether ovulation occurs or not. The pain is affected by stress, being worse when life in general is in turmoil and being eased by happy events. A D & C brings no relief, nor does the Pill, nor does a pregnancy; in fact, because it is a premenstrual symptom, it may become worse after each pregnancy. Also in contrast to spasmodic dysmenorrhea, sufferers are more mature and physically developed, with large breasts and brown nipples. An interesting fact is that smoking tends to enhance the pain associated with symptoms in the premenstruum.

Estrogen administration increases the severity of PMS, which responds positively to progesterone. On the other hand, excess progesterone administered to girls who have not borne children may rarely cause spasmodic dysmenorrhea. Thus, in theory, either type of dysmenorrhea can be produced at will by overdosing with the wrong hormone, estrogen or progesterone, which in itself proves that painful periods are not psychological but are caused by hormonal imbalances.

Despite the benefits that can be obtained by treating painful periods appropriately, certain women prefer not to ask for relief. I remember visiting a nineteen-year-old filing clerk who lived in a slum dwelling in a suburb in East London and had the flu. In conversation, her mother mentioned that her daughter also suffered from severe period pains each month and had to be brought home from the West End in a taxi. My immediate response was that suffering of this kind was no longer necessary and the pain could be treated, whereupon the girl replied, "Oh, don't! How else could I get a taxi ride once a month?"

MISPLACED CELLS

Another cause of painful periods, which may occur with the first menstruation or after years of normal menstruation, and which affects about one woman in twenty who has dysmenorrhea, is a condition known as *endometriosis*. Cells of the lining of the cavity of the womb, or endometrium, become displaced, and may be found either in the muscle wall or outer coat of the womb itself; in the ligaments around the womb; in the ovary or tubes; in the bladder or bowel; or anywhere in the lower abdomen. (Figure 34 shows the relative position of the organs around the womb.)

These cells lining the cavity of the womb have a unique ability to multiply, be shed, grow again, and multiply in an endless cycle under the influence of the menstrual hormones. Each time the lining cells of the womb are shed they pass out from the opening of the womb into the vagina and out of the body as a menstrual flow. However, the misplaced endometrial cells are not able to pass out of the body, so they tend to accumulate as tiny cysts. In time these become inflamed, covered with scar tissue and adhesions. Each time thickening of the lining occurs during the premenstruum, these cysts become larger, and as the

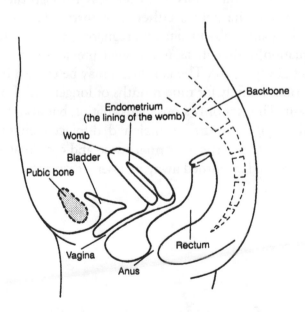

Figure 34   The position of organs around the womb

cells are shed at menstruation more room has to be found within these cysts for the extra cells. As you can imagine, over time this creates a very painful condition. The pain is not limited to the bikini area but spreads all over the lower abdomen, possibly also affecting the bladder and rectum. In addition to causing painful periods, endometriosis is usually accompanied by extreme pain during thrusting at intercourse, which may diminish all sexual desire, and also by infertility due to scar tissue forming around the ovaries and tubes. Doctors diagnose the condition by the patient's accounts of painful periods, pain at intercourse, infertility, and pain on moving the womb during a gynecological examination. If necessary they may do a laparoscopy, a keyhole surgery in which a minute periscope is inserted through a small cut in the abdominal wall, which allows the surgeon to see the tiny cysts and surrounding scar tissue.

Why the cells become displaced remains a mystery. It is possible that some were displaced during the developmental stage of the reproductive system in early fetal life. It is also possible that some lining cells find their way through the fallopian tubes into the pelvis, either at menstruation or during labor. The pain is absent during pregnancy, when there is no menstruation, although as mentioned previously, pregnancy does not always occur. The condition may be treated by stopping periods entirely for nine months or longer with hormone treatment. This not only stops menstruation but also stops the cyclical changes in the normal and displaced endometrial cells. Alternatively, the abnormal tissue and cysts may be surgically removed or burned away by laser treatment.

14

Relationships

In this chapter, the word *marriage* is used in its broadest sense—
the union of man and woman as true life partners—regardless
of whether the union was solemnized in a religious ceremony,
was legalized by being registered, or was a simple decision to
live together. This chapter is not about social conventions; it
is concerned with the effects of PMS on the lives of men,
women, and children living together as families.

Perhaps the cynic who wrote "Marriages are made in
heaven, but they end up in hell!" was married to a woman who
had a severe case of PMS. Or maybe he was just a keen observer
of other people's marriages. Not all marriages end up in hell, of
course, but for any young couple the stakes run pretty high, and
if the woman suffers from PMS or develops it later, the problems will be more intense. Most men enter relationships utterly
ignorant of the problems women face each month. The little
knowledge they have is probably confined to a vague awareness
of "periods," "bleeding," and "feminine hygiene products." If
their mothers or their sisters suffered from PMS, they might
have learned how to cope with it, but the odds are that they
paid little attention and really know very little about the cause.

Before the relationship became serious, the woman may
have avoided him on her difficult days. So, it is often not until

they are living together that the problem emerges. If she suffers from spasmodic dysmenorrhea, he will probably be the first to see that she gets effective and complete relief from her pains, for pain is something he can understand. However, sudden mood swings, irrational behavior, and bursting into tears for no apparent reason may confuse him, and sudden aggression and violence, with no warning and little justification, will shock and disturb him.

An article in the British magazine *Bride and Home* described what may lie ahead for the couple once the honeymoon is over:

Then quite suddenly you feel as if you can't cope anymore—everything seems too much trouble, the endless household chores, the everlasting planning of meals. For no apparent reason you rebel: "Why should I do everything?" you ask yourself defiantly. "I didn't have to do this before I was married. Why should I do it now?" Everything starts going wrong, and it gets worse instead of better.

As on other mornings, you get up and cook breakfast while your husband is in the bathroom. You climb wearily out of bed and trudge down the stairs, a vague feeling of resentment growing within you. The sound of cheerful whistling from upstairs only makes you feel a little more cross. Without any warning the toast starts to scorch, and the sausages, instead of happily sizzling in the pan, start spitting and spluttering furiously. Aghast, you rescue the toast, which by this time is beyond resurrection and fit only for the trash. The sausages are charred relics of their former selves and you throw those out too. Your unsuspecting husband opens the kitchen door expecting to find his breakfast ready and waiting, only to see a smoky atmosphere and a thoroughly overwrought wife. You are so dismayed at him finding you in such chaos that you just burst helplessly into tears.

What is the young husband going to make of this situation? Much depends upon his family background. If he encountered similar situations at home before marriage, he will probably react as he did then. If he is used to making himself scarce and getting out of the house, he'll probably grab his things and dash for the office, leaving his wife to sort out her troubles. If he was in the habit of helping to sort out the chaos, he'll probably sympathize with her, give her a kiss, make her a cup of coffee and breakfast, and insist on her going back to bed for the day. Obviously, this is the wisest course of action.

But what if he has never encountered this sort of thing before? How will he cope? Will he ignore it, hoping that it is only a temporary lapse until, once a month, month after month, it recurs? Or will he rage about breakfast being ruined and storm out of the house, to arrive at work hungry and unable to do his work properly, eventually returning home tired and frustrated to an equally distraught wife? Not a happy omen.

Fortunately, not all women suffer from PMS, and not all PMS sufferers become hellcats. The husband-to-be should be educated about the problems that can arise, how to recognize them, and what treatments are available to provide complete relief.

So far in this chapter we have been considering the situation of a newlywed woman with PMS. Often, however, PMS does not start until after a pregnancy. Just imagine the situation. The couple have enjoyed their life together for a year or more, until the baby came along, and now once a month there are the frustrations, mood swings, irritability, and apparent laziness—in addition to having to cope with the baby. Once, the husband could do nothing wrong; now he finds he can do nothing right on those terrible days. If he has been observant and kept track of her menstrual dates, he may soon recognize the time relationship. Realizing the importance of food, especially frequent starchy snacks, for those with PMS, they should both keep a careful eye on her eating habits. On the other hand, if neither of them has any clear idea of her menstrual dates, they will probably go on fighting month after month until they can't stand it any longer.

All this suffering is quite unnecessary and a tragic destruction of family life. The answer lies in the true nature of marriage, which is that both partners share equally in every aspect of their lives. If, when their relationship becomes serious, they both discuss the issue and keep a chart of her menstruation and any symptoms that she has, they will soon realize when things are going wrong. That is the time to seek medical advice and obtain treatment. Keeping the chart together will help them to understand each other better, and the man will have a much greater understanding of what menstruation means to a woman. He may also find that he is the first to notice the warning signs of PMS, such as a slight irrationality of conversation, or lack of conversation, and the minor disagreements in which there is a certain rigidity in her views. Another important sign is the darkening of the skin around the eyes, one of the surest signs that she is about to enter her premenstruum. In some women the skin goes so dark as to appear almost black.

If they have children, he should remember that they are more likely to get out of hand when their mother is less able to care for and play with them. He should try to be a substitute mother as well as a father, as best he can. He should remember that there is housework to be done, and it is no use telling her to rest—if the work has to be done and there is no one else to do it, she will not rest. A neighbor or a relative could be asked to help; it will probably be for only four or five days, unless the symptoms are very severe. Once menstruation has started, and while the events are still fresh in their minds, they should discuss whether she is getting adequate medical help, and he should assure her that he will support her. More husbands accompany their wives to the doctor or hospital when asking for help for PMS than for any other gynecological condition, including infertility.

The following excerpts from letters reveal how often the husband is involved with his wife's PMS:

> I am fortunate in having a very understanding husband who puts up with my tirades as best he can, but he says he sometimes doesn't know how to cope with me.

My husband first noticed the connection with my menstrual cycle without mentioning it to me eighteen months ago, and backs me up completely in writing to you.

The misery has gone on for years, misery and misery. Seventeen jobs in ten years. Now I clean offices, and for two weeks out of the month my husband gets up at 4:00 A.M. and does them for me.

Frequently, men devise their own means of confirming the diagnosis beforehand; thus the computer manager came to the clinic complete with a computer printout to prove it, while a draftsman turned up with a beautifully drawn blueprint; others merely bring along the office or kitchen calendar.

There are still too many men out there who have not made the diagnosis or who do not realize that help is available. They may know when they wake up that it's going to be one of those days, and no matter what they do, they will not be able to satisfy her. If he returns home with red roses she'll ask, "Why didn't you bring me my favorite chocolates?" But when he brings the right kind of chocolates it'll be, "You know I'm dieting, how can you be so cruel?" He just can't win.

The monthly problems can interfere with their social life and even with his earning capacity. Some years ago, a door-to-door salesman was sent by his employer for medical help. He worked on commission, and while his average weekly commission was quite high, one week in four his earnings fell drastically. Not only did he find it difficult to plan his spending, but his chances of promotion were being affected. He explained to the doctor that he became more depressed and seemed to start work later during the weeks when his earnings were low, and he could not explain why. When asked about his wife's menstruation, however, the connection dawned on him. A few days later he brought along his wife's menstrual record, which confirmed that her premenstrual irritability and tiredness were affecting him. She was delighted to be offered PMS treatment, and she responded well. Her husband was also delighted when he got a promotion.

Marital conflict is a recurring theme among those seeking medical help:

> My marriage broke up seven years ago, and I feel this trouble was a big cause of the breakup. I have since turned down a chance to remarry, as I cannot face burdening someone else with my continual monthly problems.

> This premenstrual misery is a very real threat to the survival of our marriage.

> We have been married for eight years, during which time my premenstrual tension has been a constant problem. During the past three years this has become more acute and increasingly more severe, with a traumatic effect on our relationship and on our two boys of five and three years.

> My husband has urged me to write; our marriage is breaking up, my children are suffering, and after five years of my trouble my poor husband can take no more.

> My husband has already left me, and I have two children with whom I try hard not to lose my temper at this time, but I feel sorry for them; it is really awful.

> I have come to dread my periods, and even my husband rushes to the calendar at an unexpected outburst on my part. I get violent with my husband.

Sometimes the marital disharmony just manifests as silence, on other occasions there are vicious verbal battles, and, at the extreme limit, fights and battering. How many wives batter their husbands during their paramenstruum is unknown, nor do we know how often the husband is provoked by her premenstrual anger and batters her.

One mother wrote about a daughter who was receiving treatment for premenstrual irritability and food cravings:

Some cakes and cookies I had been saving for a party disappeared on Sunday. It was all too much for me and I burst into tears. This in turn upset my husband, who went and found Mary in her bedroom and gave her a thrashing. At midnight we discovered she was missing. She had spent the night with friends. Both Mary and I started menstruating that day.

This is also a case of menstrual synchrony, in which the mother's and daughter's menstruation occurred at the same time and the mother's distress caused the husband to take it out on his daughter.

Two researchers in Washington, D.C., Roger Langley and Richard Levy, have estimated that there are twelve million battered husbands in the United States. They believe it is the "most unreported crime," affecting 20 percent of husbands. Again, one wonders how often these wives were also victims of their own hormonal imbalance.

A couple of letters suggest that the premenstruum may frequently be the cause:

I attacked him with a carving knife on one occasion, and another time while building a stone wall I lifted huge stones and threw them at him.

I have tried to knife my husband too many times to count . . . but for one fantastic week I feel on top of the world.

Most marriage counselors are well aware of the traumas that PMS can cause to the marital relationship, and they try to let the partner know about this. Often, when telephoned urgently for help because of a big fight, a wise counselor will arrange a meeting seven days later, when the woman is more likely to be in her postmenstrual phase, will have more insight, and will be more open to reason.

For most of the month, a housewife works all day in the home, dealing with the cooking, cleaning, shopping, laundry, ironing, and perhaps even the gardening. On certain days, though, it may all become too much. She may feel too apathetic to cope with the chores, may avoid the cooking, and may leave the house untidy. Alternatively, she may have a spurt of restless energy and obsessively clean and polish everything until she wears herself out. Then she may blame her premenstrual symptoms on the fact that she overdid it. One difficulty facing the woman who is at home all day is the temptation to miss meals, waiting to enjoy a meal with her husband at night.

Similarly, the working wife will run out to do the shopping during her lunch break and also miss a meal. The busier she is, the more quickly time passes, and the longer the intervals between food. During the paramenstruum this can result in the problems caused by low blood sugar levels. The woman who works away from the home also faces other problems. In an effort to control herself in front of her fellow workers, and possibly also the public, she may hold back her frustrations until she reaches home and then let go at her nearest and dearest. An important problem the couple must face is that of sexual harmony. Dr. Ruth D'arcy Hart, medical officer at the Fertility and Problems Clinic in London, found that 60 percent of married women noted that their sex urge was greatest before menstruation. Unfortunately for those with PMS, this is also the time at which many of them are least approachable, feel most unloved, and, out of anger, may refuse their husband's sexual overtures. (Incidentally, one of the side effects of the Pill that is too rarely mentioned is its ability to decrease the natural sex urge.) Satisfactory sex between partners is the best cement for any marriage. There is much that can be done these days if difficulties develop in this area, and it is really worthwhile to seek help. One cause of a decrease in sexual satisfaction, which has only recently been recognized but is most responsive to treatment, is the loss of the sex urge that occurs after a pregnancy complicated by postnatal depression. A blood test may show the wife to have a raised prolactin level, in which case treatment with bromocriptine can help.

Margaret Henderson of Australia has shown that some men have an ovulation temperature chart that is synchronous with their partners' charts. When the woman has a mid-cycle temperature drop followed by a rise at ovulation lasting for twelve to fourteen days until she menstruates, the man also has a temperature drop followed by a rise, although the temperature does not stay up. However, if the woman has an anovular cycle, with no drop and rise at ovulation, the man's chart follows hers and he does not show an ovular rise. If the woman goes on the Pill or becomes pregnant, and so stops ovulating, again the man does not have the characteristic drop and rise. If he moves out to live alone, or with another man, again the characteristic drop and rise will be lost. Although this work remains unproven, it does suggest that close companionship and harmony between a couple can lead to their bodies' rhythms becoming synchronous, with the man following the woman's cycle pattern.

As mentioned earlier, many husbands accompany their wives to the doctor's office if she is suffering from PMS, and those who don't go to the initial visit usually agree to come to the next interview. This is a most valuable opportunity for them to learn more about the full extent of their partner's problems. At the same time, much useful information can be given to them to help them to cope better. First, a husband must understand what PMS is, why it occurs, and the importance of the Three-Hourly Starch Diet. Second, he should appreciate which of his partner's symptoms can be helped, and which ones are not premenstrual but occur throughout the month and therefore are not likely to benefit from progesterone treatment. He should be taught how to chart the symptoms and may want to keep his own chart of events.

Often, the man is the first to realize that his partner could use some extra progesterone, and it may be possible to give the couple permission to raise the dose when they jointly feel it is needed. He should also understand the problems brought on by low blood sugar levels, that his partner will feel worse if she is deprived of sleep, and that during the premenstruum, her desire for alcohol may increase but she will become intoxicated on half her usual amount. If she already has a tendency toward excessive consumption of alcohol, then this is a time for him to give special care and support.

If the man really understands the situation, he will be much more able to help make the necessary adjustments to their life. Quite a few men phone home at regular intervals to ensure that their partners are eating regularly. One, aware of his wife's irritability in the premenstruum, asked the bank manager to send their joint balance sheets on specified days, so that they could discuss financial arrangements calmly in her postmenstruum. During the premenstruum, decisions about stressful things such as moving, holidays, and schools should be delayed for a week or so. If help is needed in the home, it may be better to arrange this for the one special week of the month rather than the usual one day per week.

How much responsibility should a man have for his partner's premenstrual violence? In addition to ensuring that she receives medical treatment, and providing for the care of the children and the home when she is most vulnerable, does he have a responsibility for the protection of the public? Should he report her violence to some appropriate authority? In fact, who is the appropriate authority? What are his responsibilities if her violence brings her into conflict with the law? Too often, such cases are reported too late, when the woman is already charged with assault, baby battering, or murder, and the man in her defense produces disturbing stories of her cyclical problems. All these questions need serious consideration, for at present there are no clear guidelines to help the unfortunate family in such desperate circumstances.

It is regrettable that successive cultures over the centuries have encouraged the idea that women are enigmas, with problems they must resolve themselves, and that they should just get on with it. Today we recognize that such ideas are apocryphal legacies of the past, but attitudes change slowly, and only when men have a more complete understanding of women's problems will any real progress be made.

15

※

Advice for Men

PMS is a man's problem too. With about 40 percent of women suffering from PMS, the law of averages ensures that sooner or later a man will find himself on the receiving end. It could be his mother, sister, partner, girlfriend, or any woman in his workplace or anywhere else. If he has not learned to handle the situation and doesn't know where to turn for help, then it could be a very traumatic experience indeed.

It is often said that if men suffered from PMS they would soon find a cure. Well, men do suffer from the effects of PMS in the women with whom they come in contact, either at work or at play. It has been so for thousands of years, yet they are mighty slow at recognizing it, diagnosing it, and understanding the treatment required. Usually those men who do suffer do not discuss it with other men, and therefore they feel they are dealing with an exceptional, unpredictable, or difficult woman. When they do talk to other men they are surprised to find that many have similar problems, and some are even worse off.

MALE REACTIONS

Only those who have encountered the suddenly changed personality of a woman severely affected by PMS and have come face-to-face with her unreasonableness and anger can have any idea of the accompanying trauma and sense of unreality. As the emotion of this irrational situation sweeps away common sense and reason, feelings of numbness and impotence take over. The man's thinking becomes disjointed and incoherent, and he feels powerless and immobilized by the flood of abuse that submerges his own personality, until in sheer confusion and desperation he runs away.

This situation is graphically presented in *Albert and Victoria*, David Duff's book on the married life of Queen Victoria (London: Tandem Press, 1972). It vividly portrays the reactions of Queen Victoria's husband and ministers, showing their confusion and inability to cope when faced with an irrational premenstrual outburst from a woman who was their queen but whose tension, irritability, changing moods, violence, and periods of negative attitudes were quite incomprehensible to them. They were all baffled, unsure of what they should do, and quite unable to deal effectively with the situation. The reaction of Albert, the prince consort, was to try logical arguments. Like many other men, he did not appreciate or understand the unreasoned emotion that surged like a maelstrom in Queen Victoria's brain. He did not realize that one cannot talk logic to an illogical mind, and that that is the state of the PMS sufferer at such a moment.

Even Lord Melbourne, "a past master at dealing with women," was unable to handle the situation, to say nothing of one poor cabinet minister who simply fled, too frightened to even follow the correct protocol for leaving the queen's presence. Here were three men, presumably of high intelligence, so greatly affected by their situation yet unable to take any positive action or do anything to prevent a recurrence. Who knows how many other people in the course of history have faced similar situations and not had the knowledge to do anything about them?

Ten years earlier, Charles Lamb, the great English essayist, had died. For some twenty-five years he had been at the receiving end of recurrent attacks of premenstrual violence by his sister, Mary Lamb, during one of which she killed their mother.

With great loyalty and courage Charles Lamb took upon himself the burden of responsibility for his sister's care. With her consent, he would lock her up in a special closet each month at the time of her attacks. He was rewarded with her lifelong affectionate devotion, for she kept house for him and helped with his writings, which also shows her postmenstrual normalcy.

Similar events occur daily all around us, yet most of us turn a blind eye to them. Is it not time that men decided to learn more about this disease and the way to handle it? It has been suggested that PMS is a disease of twentieth-century civilization, but this is true only to the extent that the media today exploits it, and it offers a chance for profit to quacks and entrepreneurs.

PMS has been around for thousands of years. Hippocrates in 400 B.C. suggested that it was caused by "agitated blood trying to find a way out of the body." A century earlier Simonides of Ceos, the Greek poet, wrote a classic poem about the changing moods of women, which he likened to the changing moods of the sea. This image provides an unmistakable representation of the sudden personality changes of the premenstrual woman.

MEN ARE DIFFERENT

"Why can't a woman be more like a man?" explodes Professor Higgins in *My Fair Lady*, Lerner and Lowe's musical adaptation of George Bernard Shaw's *Pygmalion*. Thousands of men must have felt like this when faced with their fair lady's attacks of PMS. Professor Higgins's outburst can be taken in two ways: either as a frustrated protest or as a serious question. Nature, having planned males and females for different functions in reproduction, has also ensured that a woman cannot behave like a man, and vice versa. Men and women are equal but different. What is more, it is impossible for a man to experience what a woman has to go through as a consequence of her role in Nature's plan. There is no way that a healthy man can have any idea of what it is like to be unable to control his actions or behavior at certain times of the month, as is the case for some women with PMS.

So what can he do to help? He needs to be aware of her problems and to be sympathetic and supportive during the pre-menstrual days. He should realize and reassure her that help is available and that there is no reason for her to suffer unnecessarily. Now that the hormonal background of PMS is becoming increasingly understood, there is so much more that can be done to control and eliminate the suffering.

RECOGNIZE THE EARLY SIGNS

Some men remain unaware of the problem until they awaken one morning to a hysterical and completely irrational woman with whom it is impossible to reason, and who may become violent. This is recognizing PMS the hard way. Others, who are more observant, may gradually become aware of her changing moods. She may become pessimistic, negative, and withdrawn at times, and at those times nothing can be done to please her. She may be snappy, argumentative, impatient, and illogical; or she may shout, shriek, yell, and swear. She may even be violent, ready to bang on the table, slam doors, throw plates, vases, and books, kick the dog or cat, or hit those nearest and dearest to her, which means her husband and children.

This emphasizes the need for keeping a menstrual chart (see page 18) to keep track of these mood changes. Frequently, it is the man in her life who first makes the connection and recognizes a woman's menstrual cyclicity. Not every PMS sufferer knows she has the disease. She may believe her mood swings are caused by an explosive personality and cannot be prevented, in which case a menstrual chart will help her to realize where the symptoms come from.

During her premenstruum, a woman may change her tastes in food, clothes, or furnishings. Her partner may return from work to find the room changed around, or in the process of being rearranged and left for him to finish. She may have food binges, alcoholic urges, and spending sprees, buying things she does not need, clothes that do not fit, and food she never eats.

Some women have "lazy" days, when they would rather not exert themselves. Others have "energetic" days, when they will not sit down and are forever tidying up and finding more jobs to do. Yet others have "urgent" days, when everything must be done today, immediately, not tomorrow or next week. No two women are alike.

A few women become paranoid during the premenstruum and accuse their partner of all sorts of outrageous behavior, often suspecting an affair. These are the "unforgetting and unforgiving" days, but they, too, will pass. Some have "jealousy" days, which recur monotonously each cycle. Until she gets treatment, it is best to accept this. Don't protest, but try not to show any interest in other women during this time. It is also no use arguing logically during the premenstruum; just wait until the postmenstruum, when she will be calmer and ready to listen—although she may then be tormented with guilt at her earlier behavior.

Perhaps the most difficult thing to understand is that just when women suffering from PMS are most unbearable is often also the time when some of them most enjoy sex. It may sound contradictory and incomprehensible, but that gives some idea of the irrationality that accompanies the hormonal upset.

How to Cope

The most important piece of advice during her difficult time: don't reason, discuss, or argue with her. Above all, keep control of yourself, and try not to become angry. Remember that PMS is an illness, a disease. Don't say, "Of course! It's the wrong time of the month!" Don't show her the menstrual chart to prove you are right. Do keep reassuring her of your concern, support, and love; she needs this, even though she may reject it. Try especially to help her to eat a little, and often. Find her favorite snacks and make sure there are plenty around. Don't worry if she has an eating binge: it is a sign that the sugar stores in her body are seriously depleted and she needs to replenish them. Instead, try to make sure it is her last binge by getting her to eat some starchy food every three hours (see chapter 24). Discourage her from starting on a weight-loss diet until her PMS has been properly treated. Admire her good qualities, and don't mention her weight or tease her about her figure. If necessary, phone her during the day to ensure that she is eating something regularly, or ask a neighbor or co-worker to check on her. If she likes alcohol, she may experience very strong urges to drink during this time, so keep an eye on the home supplies, and if they are disappearing too rapidly, then suggest removing all alcohol from the home.

Explain to your children that Mother is not well today. If possible, arrange for a neighbor, friend, or member of the family to take care of them for a day or even for a few hours. The opportunity will always arise for you to repay the kindness. Children can also be very helpful in ensuring that their mother eats regularly if you give them the necessary instructions and leave the food in a convenient place.

Use these difficult days to learn all you can about PMS. Make an appointment to see the doctor with her when she is in the postmenstruum. Doctors are often more sympathetic about PMS when the partner accompanies the patient. Remember to take the menstrual chart with you; it is the only thing the doctor needs to make a firm diagnosis. Tell the doctor how it is affecting your life as well as hers. Find out about local support or self-help groups. Many support groups encourage partners, and if your group does, then take advantage of it. You may be surprised to find that other men suffer even more than you.

If it is necessary for her to have progesterone treatment, learn all about it, and see that she takes it as instructed. If she is allowed to increase the dose when needed, then you will probably be the first to realize when that time comes. If she is a candidate for progesterone injections, consider giving them. It is not difficult to do. Many partners of diabetics give them their insulin injections.

When men learn to recognize PMS and understand how to help sufferers, then there will be no need for them to be on the receiving end. Harmony will return to the household, and women will be happier and better able to cope with their life.

16

———— ?◐ ————

Motherhood

The mother is the linchpin of the family. When her life is made miserable each month by the effects of PMS, it affects the whole family: husband, babies, schoolchildren, and teenagers. Children, even infants of only a few months, are very sensitive to changes in their mother's moods. If they cannot understand the reason for a change, they will react to it in their own peculiar way.

When you ask adult sufferers of PMS if their mothers also suffered in the same way, you are likely to get many positive—and some rather interesting—replies, such as these:

We used to say, "The dragon's on the warpath," and we all knew what it meant. But it only lasted a day or two.

I remember my brother putting up a red flag on the front door to warn us to be careful in our approach to mother.

Health professionals and social workers soon recognize when one of the mothers in their care is in her premenstruum. The usually tidy house is not picked up, the beds aren't made, dirty dishes sit on the kitchen table, and there might be a burned cake by the sink. Perhaps the children went off to school late, in yesterday's clothes, and chances are that meals will not be ready on time.

Although PMS may start at puberty, it can also begin— or get worse—after children are born. The 1983 survey of PMS women who had received progesterone noted that 57 percent of 157 women stated that their PMS increased in severity after a pregnancy. This is particularly marked in those who suffered postnatal depression or puerperal psychosis. In 1983 in San Francisco, I reported that in a survey of women who had previously suffered postnatal depression or puerperal psychosis 83 percent of three hundred women subsequently suffered from PMS, severe enough for them to seek medical help. This was a recurring theme in many letters:

> Since the birth of my last child two years ago (I have five children), I have changed from being a normal housewife and mother to an unpredictable, bad-tempered person. During my period, my moods make me feel positively ill, especially my head. If only I could grow a new one, I say to my husband.

> I have had attacks of depression since the birth of my first child, and I have never regained confidence in myself since then.

> After the baby's birth I changed, and now I get an incredible amount of head pressure for a few days prior to the bleeding. It feels as though the top of my head is about to blow off with pressure. I spoke to my doctor about the possibility of an early menopause starting, but he only smiled and said it was more likely premenstrual tension.

> I have a twenty-two-month-old son, and I cannot remember feeling like this before he was born. I love him very much, but the poor little soul does have a terrible time when I shout at him and make him sob his heart out. I seem unable to stop, although I feel terrible about

what I'm doing. It's almost as though I must be getting some sort of pleasure from it, and I feel very, very upset and guilty afterwards.

Many health professionals will agree with Dr. Christine Cooper, a pediatrician who first noticed that children can be psychologically damaged for life by verbal violence.

The sudden onset of irritability after the birth of a child may surprise many mothers, who did not experience it before. They find themselves becoming quick-tempered and making totally irrational decisions. They become impatient with the children, not waiting for them to learn to dress or eat for themselves. They become intolerant, won't accept that "kids will be kids," shout at them when they are playing harmlessly, and complain that the children won't behave. They are like the schoolteachers' helpers, who had a higher standard of discipline when they themselves were menstruating (see pages 104, 107).

When a mother has a great deal to do, it is easy for her to miss her own meals while feeding the family; alternatively, she may be dieting. Unfortunately, her irritable and aggressive outbursts are likely to occur when her blood sugar level is at its lowest, which makes matters even worse (see page 41).

Rose, an intelligent, unmarried twenty-four-year-old mother, contacted the National Society for the Prevention of Cruelty to Children, as she feared she might harm her six-year-old son during her premenstruum. It was obvious from her story that she had come very close to hurting him. She described her usual day: "Getting up at 8:00 A.M. and having a meal of toast and coffee together, then walking half a mile to his school, doing the shopping on the way home, then housework until it was time to pick him up from school at 3:30 P.M." This was the worst time of the day, and just before her periods she would feel aggressive as she met him. Suddenly a surge of hatred would well up and if he didn't behave, this is when he would be beaten.

In fact, Rose was describing how she became angry toward her son seven hours after her last meal, having expended a lot of energy during the interval. Her menstrual chart confirmed that she lost her temper only during the premenstruum. Since she has started receiving treatment and eating a midday meal and regular snacks every day, she has been happier and trouble-free. Rose also began to mark in advance on her menstrual chart the days on which she had to exert extra self-control, because she was anxious to do the best she could for her son.

Two remarks I often hear after successful treatment of a patient are "Even my children behave better" and "They don't shout so much nowadays." Some doctors even write in their files "CBB," meaning "children behaving better." In fact, children respond more quickly to their mother's improved temper than do cats or dogs, who take a long time to forget ill treatment.

Contraception often proves a problem for those with PMS, because they are liable to have side effects on the Pill. Unfortunately, tubal ligation, previously thought to be a convenient permanent solution, has been shown to reduce the blood progesterone level. If they are receiving progesterone, this can be used contraceptively (see chapter 17).

CHILDREN CANNOT UNDERSTAND

Children, who cannot understand their mother's mood swings, may react by developing psychosomatic or bodily symptoms such as a cough, runny nose, endless crying, temper tantrums, or vomiting. In my general practice, when children were brought in with such complaints, the mother was given one chart on which to record the dates of the child's symptoms and another on which to record the dates of her own menstruation. When the mothers returned with the charts after two or three months, it was surprising how often they showed clearly that the child was reacting with various ailments to the mother's mood swings. In 1966, my survey of one hundred mothers who were visiting the doctor because their children had a cough or cold showed that 54 percent of the mothers were in their paramenstruum. The children who were brought in during the mother's paramenstruum tended to be under two years old, only children, those with symptoms of less than twenty-four hours' duration, and those whose mothers were under thirty years of age. One girl was only nine months old, yet her mother brought a chart showing that each time she had menstruated in the previous three months the child had developed a cough and runny nose. A six-month-old girl with herpes (or shingles) on her knee was brought to the office by her mother, who had had recurrent premenstrual herpes on her upper lip for several years.

Another survey was carried out among children, who were admitted to the emergency room of the North Middlesex Hospital in London. The mothers of one hundred children were interviewed, and the results were very similar. In fact, 49 percent of the mothers were in their paramenstruum on the day the child was admitted. Some were admitted because of a complaint such as asthma, abdominal pain, or a temperature of unknown cause, while others had been injured in an accident. If the mother is accident-prone during her paramenstruum, the children in her care also tend to be accident-prone. If she is tired during the paramenstruum, she may not notice little Johnny running toward an oncoming car or climbing a dangerous tree, and so he will be in even greater danger then.

One day a telephone call informed me that an eighteen-month-old boy had had a high temperature and a convulsion. This was his third convulsion at intervals of three to four weeks. Inquiry revealed that it was not related to the mother's menstrual cycle but to that of his nanny, who had total care of the boy while his mother worked full time. There had been some trouble with the nanny the day before, and she had just given notice. The two previous convulsions had occurred at the time of the nanny's paramenstruum.

SIBLING JEALOUSY

Sometimes a situation is incorrectly diagnosed as jealousy of a brother or sister, when the real diagnosis is PMS in the mother.

Susan, thirty years old, had felt very well during her second pregnancy, with plenty of energy, so she would take three-year-old David out each afternoon to play on the swings or kick a ball around in the nearby park. She had an easy delivery of a much-wanted daughter, but afterward she became so depressed that she needed psychiatric treatment. David had been dry since the age of sixteen months, but after his sister's birth he gradually started to wet the bed again, not every night, but in batches every few weeks. It seemed easy to blame it on jealousy of the new baby, but when Susan kept a careful record it showed that David's bedwetting was occurring during her premenstruum. Susan admitted that she "hadn't been the same" since the baby's birth, and had been too tired and busy to take David for his usual playtime in the park.

The most tragic aspect of PMS is when it becomes so severe that the mother, in a state of confusion and rage, batters her beloved child. These mothers, contrary to popular belief, are women who often really love their children. They have strong maternal feelings, but in a sudden moment of premenstrual irritability they lose control and harm their offspring.

A social worker's report on a thirty-five-year-old mother of two children reads:

> During the last premenstruum her youngest daughter, aged eighteen months, was screaming and would not stop. Patient was very irritated by this and picked her up and squeezed her—this started a circle of louder screaming and harder squeezing until patient "heard something crack." She was immediately frightened and threw the child on the floor and sat crying on the chair. When more composed, she examined Joan and took her to the doctor.

This type of injury to a child is, tragically, not uncommon. Judging from the letters and stories of my patients, the cases of baby battering that are reported are only the tip of the iceberg.

> Because I lost my temper and hit my eldest child when he was four, just before a period, I nearly had a complete

nervous breakdown. Even though I feel much better now, my premenstrual tension remains, and from day eighteen of the cycle until day four of my period I suffer from depression, temper, forgetfulness, and dizziness.

It has gotten to a stage now that every month something the children do triggers me off. It is as though there is somebody inside me saying terrible things. I blame my son and tell him I hate him, and hit him. Sometimes he gets out of my way quickly.

If the situation becomes worse, the children may be taken into care, but this is a drastic step. One wonders about the aftereffects on the many slightly battered children who are not referred to social services and are not helped. Does the unsettled, temperamental background of such a childhood leave scars, such as shyness or lack of confidence?

A woman who had been treated with progesterone for seventeen years was asked if she would like to take part in a television program dealing with PMS (see *Loretta*, page 257). She went home and explained to her family that she couldn't recall those far-off days. "You must be joking! Dad and I will never be able to forget your vicious temper" was the comment from her daughter, now in her twenties.

A thirty-five-year-old teacher married to the principal of a school stated,

> For seven days during the premenstruum I become tense, irritable, shouting, weepy and tired, bloated with swelling of my legs and ankles, and with headaches over my eyes. I have two children and at those times when I am in an uncontrollable temper, I have hit them really hard.

She was successfully treated with progesterone for twelve months and has been free from symptoms since. She later wrote,

> It has been a valuable experience—I would never have believed that an intelligent woman like me, with high

morals and a good education, could ever lose control of herself to such an extent that she would batter her children, for I love my children dearly. How utterly illogical it is that I personally should cause them permanent harm.

When the child reaches school, the teacher may notice that absences seem to occur at regular intervals. One ten-year-old girl was referred for treatment by her teacher, who noticed absences for a few days at the beginning of each month. The teacher wondered if it was because of the girl's menstruation, but, in fact, it was because her mother had recurrent premenstrual asthma requiring rest in bed, and the daughter was kept at home to answer the door.

TEENAGERS' REACTIONS

Truancy from school may also be related to a mother's premenstrual symptoms, as in the case of one mother, who wrote,

> For days before a period starts I hate everyone and make the family's life a misery. My thirteen-year-old daughter will not go to school when I'm like this. She is frightened of what I may do, and cries when I start drinking.

Teenagers, both boys and girls, are quick enough to spot the changes in their mothers and notice when "she's in one of those moods." As one boy put it, "Our whole life revolves around Mom's periods."

The mother's problem is not helped when the daughter starts to menstruate, especially if both periods occur synchronously. Many mothers, recognizing the problem in themselves, seek help for their daughters' PMS. They may feel that they have weathered the storm so far, and it will not be long before the end, but they are not prepared to let their daughters suffer as they have done.

All mothers—and fathers too—have the responsibility of seeing that their children receive a good sex education, especially about those problems that come back once a month.

17

❦

PMS and Contraception

It is difficult to believe that in the 1940s, medical students knew that treatment with estrogen and progestogens would cause infertility, as well as curing dysmenorrhea and regulating menstruation, and therefore its use was limited to single women and widows. It was thought that conception for married women was natural, and doctors should not interfere with Nature. Doctors appeared oblivious to the colossal, worldwide desire to limit reproduction. Marie Stopes clinics did teach occlusive contraception using the diaphragm or condom, but they treated only married women and engaged couples, who were required to bring evidence of marriage within six weeks.

Today, contraception is almost synonymous with the Pill, which is the best-known contraceptive and is widely used because of heavy promotion by multinational pharmaceuticals, to whom it is highly profitable. However, contraception is a problem for PMS sufferers, who are liable to develop side effects on the Pill, and if they choose the permanent solution of tubal ligation, their PMS is likely to increase in severity. Fortunately, there is a solution to their problem: progesterone therapy can be tailored to include contraception.

HORMONAL CONTRACEPTION

Unfortunately, too many PMS sufferers cannot manage hormonal contraception without developing unwanted side effects. The reason for this is easily explained. Hormonal contraception relies on progestogens, which lower the progesterone blood level. This was demonstrated in the 1982 survey of 614 well-diagnosed PMS sufferers.

Side Effects of Pill in 614 PMS Sufferers

- Depression, 21%
- Headache, 20%
- Weight gain, 13%
- Nausea, 10%
- Increased tension, 7%
- Bloatedness, 5%
- Loss of libido, 4%
- Breast tenderness, 3%

There are numerous different types of hormonal contraception, including the conventional estrogen/progestogen pill, as well as biphasic, triphasic, and everyday combined pill, progestogen only, and long-acting injections and implants, such as Norplant. All types are badly tolerated by PMS sufferers, although most try changing to different brands before stopping this method of contraception completely.

Furthermore, PMS sufferers are more likely to suffer from the downside of the Pill, with complications such as deep vein thrombosis, pulmonary embolism, strokes, and coronary disease. Progesterone is required by the endothelial cells, those innermost cells of blood vessels, which ensure that blood flows smoothly (see pages 76, 91). The risks of these side effects are greatest among smokers.

The reaction to the inability to tolerate the Pill because of side effects varies with individuals, depending on their knowledge of the subject and realization that it is a risk factor for PMS. The examples of Myra and Tiffy show different

reactions, although both lived in the same leafy London suburb, both were aged thirty-five at the time of their first consultation, and both were the eldest child in a family of two.

Myra tried the Pill during her first year away at college;
she realized within the first week that she became depressed
and unexpectedly rude and insolent. She stopped taking the
Pill and after six weeks tried another lower-dose one, but the
same problems arose, so she accepted that the Pill was not for
her and changed to a diaphragm. She became a successful
lawyer and married at the age of twenty-eight. Her health had
always been excellent. Their first child was planned and she
remained well during pregnancy, working until four weeks
before the easy birth of her son. Then the unexpected happened: she developed postnatal depression and became anxious, miserable, insecure, and flat over the next few weeks. She
tried the Pill, but immediately her depression became worse.
She needed and sought psychiatric help, and was rescued by
psychiatric medication. Life returned to normal except for the
premenstrual week, when all her usual miseries returned. Myra
was ultimately treated with progesterone and the Three-
Hourly Starch Diet. She is using the diaphragm again.

Tiffy was accompanied on her first consultation by her
mother, who immediately admitted she was a sufferer of PMS and
had been treated for it. She told me her daughter's sad tale. When
Tiffy had her first menstruation at fourteen, it had been accompanied by an extraordinary outburst resulting in her breaking her
bedroom mirror, but subsequently her periods were normal. At
sixteen, to keep up with her peers, she started taking the Pill.
This changed her into an aggressive, argumentative, and violent
girl. Her mother suspected the Pill, but Tiffy would not listen and
refused to stop taking it. No longer could there be any calm discussions with her mother, father, or younger sister. She hated herself and everyone, including her teachers, so although one of the
brightest students, she left school and home and drifted away, no
one knew where. On three occasions during the next two years,
calls from distant hospitals informed the parents that she had

been admitted following an overdose. Although the parents traveled miles to see her, she refused to return home. After she had been absent for ten years, the parents learned that Tiffy was detained and sectioned in a mental hospital for causing a street disturbance while dancing naked under the influence of alcohol. She was started on psychiatric medication and the Pill was stopped. This time, when Tiffy was discharged after six months she agreed to return home. Although she was sedated by psychiatric medication, her mother recognized the underlying PMS, which was treated while gradually reducing and finally stopping all other prescribed medication. She has returned to college and is trying to make up her lost years.

These cautionary tales suggest that teachers and counselors should be aware of the behavior-altering effect of hormonal contraception on a few unlucky individuals.

Dr. Riddoch and her team in Tasmania studied the effect of the Pill on 227 attendees at the Family Planning clinic. They noted that the single most common side effect was weight gain, and they recommended counseling about diet when they start women on the Pill.

It must be appreciated that those who have difficulty in tolerating the Pill are also likely to have difficulty at the menopause with estrogen replacement therapy (ERT), which also contains estrogens and progestogen, although at a lower dose.

PROGESTERONE CONTRACEPTION

Progesterone is as effective as the progestogen-only pill and the intrauterine device. Low-dose progesterone is given vaginally or rectally from Day 8 until menstruation, although progesterone users will increase to their normal progesterone dosage from ovulation to menstruation.

Many who are already using two or more suppositories of 400 mg may prefer to cut a 400 mg suppository in half and use 200 mg daily in the follicular phase—it is just as effective. Figure 35 shows the dose used in studies in 1987 and 1992.

Progesterone Contraception for PMS

Daily low-dose (100 or 200 mg)
progesterone suppository from Day 8 of the cycle.

Increase to optimum progesterone dosage at ovulation.

Continue daily progesterone until menstruation.

Starting progesterone early may stimulate growth of the lining of the womb (the endometrium) and result in slight bleeding or early menstrual bleeding. The answer is to use the lowest dose of 100 mg on Day 8 and continue on that dose until two days after ovulation, when the full progesterone dose can be used. Some women prefer to use a condom (male or female variety) or diaphragm until two days after they have started their normal PMS progesterone course from ovulation to menstruation.

A study reported at the 1994 Dalton Society meetings in London of 253 severe PMS sufferers using progesterone contraception showed 15 failures over an average of 5.82 years. This means a failure rate of 2.66 per 100 women/years (Figure 36). Women/years is the usual method of measuring contraceptive effectiveness, and refers to 100 women using a method for one year, or 50 women using it for two years, and so on. The failure rate of the condom is reckoned as 14, diaphragm as 12, rhythm method as 24, and intrauterine device as 2.3 women/years. In the reported study the failure rate was mostly due to patient failure, such as forgetting to take the contraceptive, especially when traveling, starting too late, or a bout of diarrhea. Incidentally if diarrhea occurs, the suppository can still be used vaginally.

TUBAL LIGATION

Once the family is complete, and because there are unpleasant side effects from hormonal contraception, a permanent solution would appear to be closure of the two fallopian tubes. It can be done very simply with clips, clamps, sutures, cautery, or

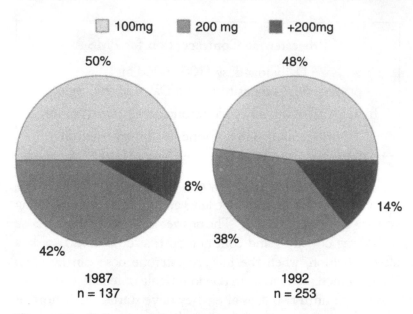

Figure 35   Follicular dose of progesterone for contraception

cutting away portions of the tube. Unfortunately, it matters not which method is used to ensure the tubes are blocked, as all methods seem to increase the subsequent PMS, and in addition there may be pain with menstruation or heavy bleeding. This is something gynecologists rarely warn their patients about in their preoperative consultation, but it is commonly observed.

Exactly why there is this increase in severity of PMS after sterilization is a frequent topic of medical conversation. It may be because the ovarian nerve, artery, and vein are closely attached to the fallopian tubes as they pass from the womb to the ovaries, and they may also be blocked. Radwanksi, Hammond, and Berger showed in 1979, and it has since been confirmed, that following tubal ligation there is a lower output of progesterone from the ovaries. It may possibly be related to progesterone receptors, for it is known that the level of progesterone receptors in the tubes is very high.

An interesting observation, not yet confirmed, is that women who have tubal ligation before the age of thirty-five

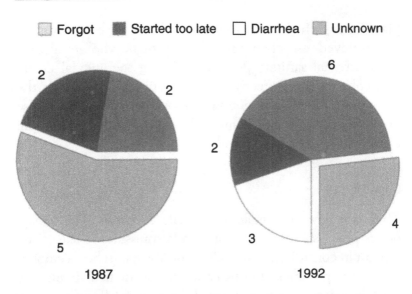

Figure 36   Reasons for failures of progesterone contraception

tend to have a low bone mineral density at the age of fifty. This means they are more likely to develop osteoporosis in later life.

INTRAUTERINE DEVICE

The intrauterine device is suitable for those who have had a pregnancy and are free from pelvic infection. The usual reason for removal of the device is either period pain or heavy bleeding. To overcome the problem of heavy bleeding, a device called Mirena has been developed, which contains a very low dose progestogen. In theory, this might interfere with the progesterone blood level and increase PMS, but it is still too early to report on its side effects.

DIAPHRAGM AND CERVICAL CAP

The diaphragm and cervical cap are both useful methods of contraception, which depend on the reliability of the patient. They need to be available when required and should be left in place for eight hours after intercourse. They are easily inserted and removed, especially for today's women, who are already using internal sanitary protection. Using spermicidal cream may enhance their effectiveness. It should not be used at the same time as a progesterone suppository, because the wax base of the suppository may damage the fabric of the diaphragm, causing minute holes to develop.

CONDOMS

There are now both male and female condoms. The female one is safer as it does not burst under pressure. It leaves the woman in control. British health education in schools emphasizes the importance of using condoms for the first six months of each new relationship to avoid the risk of AIDS.

MORNING-AFTER MEDICATION

When there has been unprotected sex and conception is unwanted, then high-dose estrogen and progestogen taken within seventy-two hours may abort a possible pregnancy. Four tablets of Schering PC4 are the only licensed post-coital medication in Britain (they are not available in the United States). Two tablets are taken as soon as possible within seventy-two hours and a further two tablets after twelve hours. Nausea and vomiting within two hours of either dose are common side effects, and if vomiting occurs an extra two tablets should be taken. It is recognized that vomiting impairs the efficiency. Unfortunately, it is sufferers of PMS who are most likely to develop vomiting. More than one PMS sufferer has preferred the option of termination of the possible pregnancy to another course of post-coital medication.

18

---- ❧ ----

Women at Work and Play

The cost to industry because of menstrual problems is high and is measured in millions of pounds, liras, kroners, and dollars, as well as in terms of human misery, unhappiness, and pain. It has been estimated to cost U.S. industry 8 percent of its total wage bill, compared with 5 percent in Sweden, 3 percent in Italy, and 3 percent in Britain. The load is not spread evenly, for the industries that suffer most are those employing large numbers of women, especially the clothing industry, light engineering, transistor and assembly factories, and laundries. Texas Instruments, which employs women for the assembly of electrical components, finds that the average worker's normal production rate of one hundred components per hour drops during the paramenstruum to seventy-five per hour.

Studies have shown that during the paramenstruum there is a deterioration of arm and hand steadiness, which is an adverse factor among those whose work demands manual dexterity. One podiatrist, who complained that during the paramenstruum her hands get stiff and she finds skilled movements difficult, said, "If I ever cut a patient, I'm sure it will be during those premenstrual days."

Absenteeism directly related to menstrual problems is generally caused by spasmodic dysmenorrhea, premenstrual migraine, and asthma. Other premenstrual symptoms are seldom considered a good enough reason to stay home, for, as one library assistant remarked,

> You don't stay away from work merely because of your bad temper. Instead, you soldier on and cause chaos by misfiling, and you get yourself a bad name.

The influence of menstrual illness during working hours was demonstrated in a survey at a light-engineering factory in North London employing 3,500 women, and also in the branches of a department store employing 10,000 women. It showed that 45 percent of the 269 women surveyed who reported sick were in their paramenstruum. Dr. William Bickers and Maribelle Woods from the Medical College of Virginia noted as long ago as 1951 that 36 percent of women in their premenstrual week requested sedation during working hours.

Twenty years ago, a survey in four London hospitals showed that half of all emergency admissions of women to hospitals occurred during the premenstruum. These findings have since been confirmed worldwide. This figure was the same for medical emergencies (like coronaries and strokes), for surgical admissions (like colic and appendicitis), for infectious fevers, and for admissions to psychiatric wards. Admissions for depression and suicides have been shown the world over to be highest during the paramenstruum.

Accidents at work are another problem to industry—both the minor cuts and bruises, which are a waste of working time and are treated at the first-aid station, and the serious ones, which require admission to the hospital. Research at the U.S. Center for Safety Education showed that the forty-eight hours before the onset of menstruation are the most dangerous ones, when most accidents occur. In Germany it was noted that apprentice tightrope walkers had the most accidents in the premenstruum. In restaurants it is recognized that the premenstrual clumsiness of waitresses accounts for an undue number of breakages.

Lowered mental ability during the paramenstruum also accounts for many unnecessary typing errors. More than one secretary has been referred for treatment when her boss could no longer put up with those few days every month when letters had to be repeatedly returned for retyping. Journalists, artists, and authors find this a problem too, lacking inspiration during this time and waiting hopefully for a brainstorm, which is more likely to come during the postmenstruum. Errors in billing, accounting, stocktaking, and filing take longer to correct than to make, and again, the incidence of mistakes is highest during the paramenstruum. Premenstrual irritability may show itself in bad-tempered service by salespeople, receptionists, and waitresses, who are all in the public view. The problems of lowered judgment during the premenstruum must be considered by teachers, judges, and executives, who need to be on their guard against making hasty and wrong decisions. One teacher wrote with honesty,

> Every month there are one or two days when I am simply not worth the salary my employers pay me.

Certain specialized occupations have their own particular hazards on premenstrual days. An example is the hoarseness that affects opera and other professional singers. One musical comedy star in the 1930s would, with devastating regularity, come into the theater once a month surrounded by a powerful aroma of garlic, which preceded her wherever she went. "You see," she would explain, "it's this sore throat again, and garlic is the only thing that saves my voice." Sure enough, four days later she would once again be in magnificent voice, but whether it was the garlic or her postmenstruum that was responsible is a matter of guesswork.

For artists in the theater, PMS is a very real problem. One great impresario always attended rehearsals wearing a top hat and smoking a cigar. On one occasion his leading lady was making a fuss and was obviously in her premenstruum. The great man stood up in the center of the auditorium, ground his cigar to dust under his feet, and hurling his hat on the floor, stamped on it, crying out, "Woman! I don't know why I employ you—you drive me to distraction!" There was a pause and in a changed voice he went on, "But when you are well, you're magnificent!"

One wonders how many so-called prima donnas, with their reputation for throwing tantrums, were really only reacting to their PMS. For the members of the chorus, the showgirls, and ballet dancers, it is always a question of whether the stage manager has enough experience to recognize their problem and help them over the difficult days. Their symptoms of bloating and puffy eyes and skin are shared by models and movie stars, who often have a clause in their contracts forbidding filming during their paramenstruum. A lowered sensitivity to taste is a handicap to cooks, who may overflavor sauces and other foods. And we should remember the Russian woman astronaut Valentina Tereshkova, who in 1973 had to be brought down after only three days in space when she began to menstruate heavily in zero gravity.

In Argentina, women are allowed under the constitution to take the necessary days off if they have menstrual problems. In India, wives have long had the privilege of being excused from housework during this time, as it is believed that any food they prepare may be spoiled.

The site of an individual's premenstrual symptoms may be related to her work. In a study of PMS carried out in a light-engineering factory, about twenty women were interviewed in batches each day. Some days it was noted that the predominant symptom was premenstrual backache; on other days, complaints of headaches were the most common. Later, it became clear that all the women in any one batch came from the same department and were doing the same kind of work. Those who spent their working hours stooped over a workbench were more likely to complain of backache, while those who sat at a bench assembling small electrical parts, a task requiring considerable concentration, mostly complained of premenstrual headaches.

Texas Instruments found that women had less menstrual absenteeism when they worked from 2:00 P.M. to 10:00 P.M., compared with the other shifts of 6:00 A.M. to 2:00 P.M. and 8:30 A.M. to 5:30 P.M. Maybe this was because if they woke up feeling ill, they had more time to take medicine and recover from their problems. It is certainly worth considering for those who are given an option to choose their own working hours. PMS sufferers usually cope especially badly with night-shift work, which seems to be because the diurnal clock, which regulates the sleep-wakefulness cycle, is situated in the hypothalamus and easily disturbs the menstrual clock. This is found to be a problem with nurses, especially those in training, whose regulations demand a specified period of night work. In November 1993 at an international congress entitled "Women, Work and Health" held in Barcelona, Wendy Holton and I reported the results of a survey on the effect of night work compared to day work on 310 PMS sufferers. The night workers, working either evening shifts or full nights, suffered more from depression, irritability, tiredness, headache, bingeing, breast tenderness, and violence. In every case, violence was directed against the partner. In addition, 54 percent also directed their violence against property—especially dishware, books, furniture, and cars—but fortunately, violence against children was the lowest.

PMS syndrome can affect a woman's chances of getting employment, holding down a job, and receiving a promotion—or losing it unnecessarily. The problems of some sufferers are shown in the following excerpts from letters:

> I cannot plan to go anywhere during these depressing times and I live in constant fear of losing my job, as I have to take time off each month with a real sick headache. My chances of promotion have been ruined because of this.

> I recently gave up my job unnecessarily, and realized that it is ridiculous to let this condition ruin my whole life.

Although I know the cause of my depressive feelings, I seem to be unable to think logically, and though I know I'll be fine again in a week, I get quite illogical and irrational at the same time.

I am thirty-three now and have suffered from PMS for the best part of my adult life. The symptoms are horrible depression, muddle-headedness, and feeling dead from the neck up. I recently took the totally unnecessary and very impulsive step of resigning from my job as an English teacher. Of course I took this drastic step just before my period. I am well qualified and have been doing this now for seven years. To all other people I appear cheerful, calm, and efficient, especially when a period is not close.

A different and very specialized hazard faced both male and female employees in the Ortho Pharmaceuticals oral contraceptive plant in Puerto Rico, where breast enlargement was found among the men and menstrual disorders among the women. This occurred despite the strict precautions taken in making the synthetic estrogens used in the contraceptives. These included hermetically sealed machines, air conditioners, respirators, and special protective clothing (even down to the underwear). The long-term effects of occupational exposure to estrogens are practically unknown, and there are no safety standards in force anywhere.

How can industry best cope with the financial burden caused by menstrual problems? Fortunately, many employers now have convenient restrooms where a woman can relax for a few hours, take something to ease her trouble, and return to continue her work. The availability of flextime, where each worker clocks herself in and out at times that suit her best, is a blessing to many women. They can accumulate a few hours' reserve, so that when they are at their lowest they need not go to work at all.

But more is needed. Industry could tackle the situation better by educating staff, especially personnel managers and supervisors, to recognize and fully understand the problems so that they can deal with them better. For example, women can be assigned to less-skilled jobs such as packing and stacking during their vulnerable days, rather than remaining on tasks that are more complex and harder to correct later, such as soldering or assembly.

Some enlightened organizations arrange talks on PMS for their workers and managers and ensure that there are nearby facilities for treatment. These treatment centers should be available either in hospitals or at places of employment.

Even when a woman is away from the office and housework and just relaxing, the black cloud of once-a-month problems may still be with her. What woman looking forward to a weekend of fun on a yacht or hiking in the mountains, on a bicycle or spelunking down in the caves, wants to be bothered with menstrual problems? Fortunately, something can be done for those women who are on the Pill. They can be asked when they start their initial course, "Which day of the week would it be most convenient for you to menstruate?" As menstruation can be expected to start within two days of stopping the course, it is not very difficult to calculate which day to begin. Of course, some women would find it more convenient to menstruate on the weekends, when their husbands can take over some domestic chores and care for the children.

SPORTS

The strenuous physical training and weight regulation demanded of top sportswomen often leads to delayed menarche, amenorrhea, infrequent and scanty menstruation, failure to ovulate, or infertility. It is now realized that it may even cause a lowering of bone mineral density, increasing the risk of osteoporosis. These symptoms occur particularly in younger athletes, and those with a low body weight and low fat percentage, especially runners, gymnasts, and ballet dancers. When amenorrhea is present, menstruation, and sometimes also ovulation, may return when training is stopped because of vacations or injuries. Intensive physical activity can delay menarche if the activity is begun before puberty. Frisch noted that among athletes who started training before their menarche, the mean age of starting menstruation was 15.1 years, compared with athletes starting training after the menarche, who had an average menarcheal age of 12.8 years.

There is a positive correlation between these menstrual problems in athletes and the intensity of their training programs. Feicht and his colleagues showed that whereas only 6 percent of athletes running less than ten miles weekly had amenorrhea, the figure rose to 43 percent for those running seventy miles or more weekly. Although superficially it may seem beneficial to be free of the hazards of menstruation or fear of pregnancy, it is now becoming clear that the attendant lack of estrogen and progesterone can result in brittle bones, as in postmenopausal women. So these young athletes become prone to stress fractures, especially of the metatarsal bones of the feet. Some studies on amenorrheic runners have shown that their bone mineral content was equivalent to that of the average fifty-two-year-old woman, which suggests that they have an urgent need for calcium and hormonal supplementation to prevent premature osteoporosis.

What about the other sporting activities that women enjoy? Those who play tennis, golf, or racquetball may find that their performance deteriorates during the paramenstruum. It has been found that during this time arm and hand steadiness is impaired, sharpness of vision declines, and movement is slower because of extra weight and water retention. The menstrual influence on top sportswomen may be less obvious because they are able to maintain a steady standard with fewer fluctuations in performance. Since the mid-seventies, however, when research by the British Women's Amateur Athletic Association confirmed that top women athletes gave their best performances during their postmenstruum, trainers have started to do a little menstrual engineering, adjusting the time of menstruation so that the athletes do not have to rely entirely on Nature's roulette.

Doctors Moller-Neilsen and Hammar from Sweden confirmed that women soccer players were more susceptible to injuries during their premenstruum and menstrual period than during the rest of the cycle, especially those with premenstrual symptoms of irritability, bloating, or breast discomfort. Fewer injuries occurred among those using oral contraceptives.

Dr. Ken Dyer of Adelaide, Australia, has produced some interesting figures showing that over the past twenty years women's top athletic performances have improved more than men's. This suggests that within the next three or four decades women could be running and swimming as well as men, certainly in the longer-distance races. Women have determination and aggression and are especially suited to prolonged exertion; there is the striking example of Canadian Cynthia Nicolas, who in the summer of 1977 set a new world record for crossing the English Channel twice in 19 hours and 55 minutes, compared with the previous male record of 30 hours.

HOBBIES

Women have many hobbies, and it is difficult to cover them all. There are those who enjoy dressmaking but know better than to cut a dress out of expensive material on the wrong day of the month in case they spoil it. Others hesitate to buy flowers at that time, as they find they cannot arrange them to their satisfaction. Artists often have difficulties or feel their inspiration is lost, and have to wait until their postmenstrual peak to resume creative activity.

Intellectual games may also be affected once a month, as the partner at bridge or the opponent at chess or Scrabble may have discovered.

DRIVING HAZARDS

Driving is more necessary than recreational for most women, but for some it may be a sport or a social activity. A few may race cars, and many take car trips, alone or with their families. In any case, there will be a menstrual handicap. A survey at four hospitals showed that half of all accident admissions of women occurred during their paramenstrual days. In fact, among those involved in an accident, the menstrual influence was equally present among the passengers—the passive participants—and the drivers—the active participants. In the few seconds between a car climbing a curb and hitting a wall an alert passenger may brace herself and cover her head for protection, but the passenger in her paramenstruum may be too slow to take even these elementary precautions.

Driving is a complicated task, requiring the coordination of many skills, which are slower during the paramenstruum. Complicated and rapidly changing road situations demand quick reactions and good judgment, and if these are impaired, problems could result, such as an increase in braking distance. Acuteness of hearing is dulled, so that a driver may not hear a warning siren. A decreased sharpness of vision and a lowered ability to judge shapes and sizes may cause a woman to lose her normal precision in parking and reversing. She may become impatient with the slow driver ahead or with an elderly person crossing the road. She may overtake dangerously, or drive aggressively around a blind corner. She may fail to notice changing weather and light conditions or alterations of the road surface. She may forget to fasten her safety belt or to follow other driving laws. Even as a pedestrian, she is more vulnerable in her paramenstruum, and she may cross the road without the usual precautions. As a mother, she may not be alert enough to protect her child from dangers on the road.

Having said all this, perhaps I should add that women are considered better risks than men are by insurance companies. Though some women are at risk during the paramenstruum, they are much safer drivers during the postmenstrual peak.

SHOPPING

The normal joys of a shopping spree may be ruined during the paramenstruum. A woman may become an indecisive, hesitant shopper who tries on all the shoes in the shop, finds they won't fit her swollen feet, and leaves empty-handed. She may buy totally inappropriate dresses that don't fit and are the wrong color, and which she will never wear. It is possible that her color sense and appreciation of shape and size deteriorate during this phase of the cycle. A few women even buy unnecessary and expensive items, like cars and jewelry. One woman in Arizona in two consecutive premenstruums bought two full-length mink coats, which she didn't need and could not really afford. One can't help feeling sorry for the man who wrote,

> I know it's the wrong day of the month for my wife if I come home and find the kitchen loaded with fruit, anything up to ten pounds of apples, bananas and oranges. I know she'll be in a terrible mood, and will ask me to put the children to bed. . . . But at other times she's the best wife in the world.

There is also the problem of women shoplifters who are caught during their paramenstruum. While it is possible that a few of them really are in a confused state and are unaware of what they are doing, others are habitual shoplifters who were caught because they were not quick enough or did not take their usual precautions.

ENTERTAINMENTS

Social entertainments may not be too successful during the paramenstruum. Cocktail parties too often require prolonged standing, which is no fun for those with water retention. As one woman put it,

I can always recognize fellow sufferers, as they also edge their way toward the walls to rest their legs.

Other problems related to this time of the month are described in the following letters:

My problem starts about ten days before my period comes. I get uncontrollable fits of depression, which make me hit rock bottom. If I'm with a crowd of friends, I feel like I'm going to suffocate; it's a feeling that just sweeps over me and I want to run out, and I do run out.

I often have to entertain for my husband. I am a good cook, even if I say so myself. I get an excellent meal ready, but when the first guest arrives I just burst into tears. It ruins my whole evening. I've learned to arrange the dates so that they come after my period, but then my period is bound to be late!

Even the theater may not bring pleasure to everyone, as one sufferer from premenstrual depression recalled:

I remember sitting in the theater with tears rolling down my cheeks, squeezing my hands and saying to myself, "No —I mustn't, this is a comedy—everyone else is laughing."

The problems of alcohol intoxication are increased during the paramenstruum, so that a woman can never really let herself go without getting into trouble. Some women can never use cannabis without suffering its worst effects, while others can use it at most times of the month and enjoy the experience. However, if they smoke it during the paramenstruum they may develop delusions or hallucinations.

Some women have an uncontrollable urge to gamble during the premenstruum, whether it is on horses, cards, or bingo. One of my patients is addicted to slot machines. Some days she is just spellbound by them and cannot stop. Now that she realizes the cause of her habit, she tries to go out without any money at those times of the month.

VACATIONS

Vacations are not always as much fun as anticipated—in fact, sometimes they are complete disasters. Flights may be delayed, so that eating schedules are completely thrown off. Women should bear this in mind when packing their carry-on luggage and keep a supply of emergency rations with them. Remember that food is not served on the plane immediately after departure, or when the plane is circling its destination for what seems like hours before receiving permission to land. Hotels in other countries may have fixed hours for meals with no arrangements for mid-morning, mid-afternoon, or late-night snacks.

Avoid night travel as much as possible, as this disturbs the day/night rhythm center in the hypothalamus, which is close to the menstrual control center. PMS sufferers are likely to have trouble with jet lag for the same reason. After a long flight, they should go straight to bed regardless of the time of day, avoiding the temptation to do some quick sightseeing or to chat with friends. A few hours' rest will do wonders to prevent the terrible lethargy that results from jet lag and can last for days.

19

❧

PMS Goes to Court

It was a surprising coincidence that in 1980, two women, each from a different city, appeared in court on consecutive days, each charged with murder, and both had their charge reduced to manslaughter on the grounds of diminished responsibility by reason of PMS. Although the circumstances of the two women's offenses differed, the evidence in both cases led to the same conclusion. Both cases had been carefully researched and presented indisputable evidence of longstanding, bizarre, cyclical behavior occurring in the premenstruum, with normal behavior in the postmenstruum.

It is important to keep in mind that these were two extreme and exceptional cases. Not all sufferers of PMS are potential murderers, nor do all female murderers suffer from PMS (see Julia, pages 257–258). The International Symposium on Premenstrual, Postpartum and Menopausal Mood Disorders held in Kiawah Island, South Carolina, in 1987, confirmed that the number of cases of severe PMS of the type described in these legal defenses and sensationalized in the press is extremely small. Yet although PMS is not yet accepted in American law, during the intervening years there have been several more PMS-related cases of murder, not so spectacular, and since that time PMS has been accepted in

English law in mitigation for most other offenses in the criminal and family court.

This legal ruling recognizing PMS places a new responsibility on the medical professions. Doctors are now frequently asked to produce for the courts their medical notes to confirm a defendant has visited them for the treatment of PMS. A recent British newspaper report read,

> A BT executive, who attacked a man in a fit of road rage, walked from court with a fine yesterday after blaming her anger on tablets that she was prescribed for premenstrual tension. J.S., 34 years, repeatedly slapped cyclist C. in the face and punched him on the chest after he banged on her new Fiat with his plastered broken arm. When then a woman police officer intervened, she slapped the man again and said to the officer "or what, you'll nick me?" . . . The defense lawyer said she had been suffering after being prescribed a course of tablets called Duphaston (a progestogen), which are used to ease PMS. She had a very bad time on these tablets. She became very irritable and bad tempered . . . since the attack she has been taken off Duphaston and put on Prozac to which she responded favorably.

It is now the duty of both the legal and the medical professions to ensure that the plea of PMS will not be abused, and that any such plea adheres to the strict definition of PMS (see chapter 2). This requires the diagnosis of PMS (see chapter 3) to be substantiated with evidence in every case, and the condition must respond to treatment. There must be evidence of recurrent symptoms; earlier episodes of a similar loss of control, confusion, or amnesia; or violence in previous cycles or at monthly intervals. Women facing charges of shoplifting are often referred to me by their lawyers, who hope to use PMS as a defense. I first give them the definition of PMS and then ask,

"What did you steal in the last two months, before your menstruation?" This is usually enough of a shock, and most of them leave the consulting room hurriedly, muttering, "But this really is my first offense . . ." Even if it is their first occasion of shoplifting, a PMS patient should be able to recall previous episodes when she has been forgetful, confused, or disoriented, and an effort should be made to find evidence of a relationship of such episodes to menstruation.

FACTUAL EVIDENCE

The necessary evidence, if it is there, may be found in diaries, medical records, police files, or prison documents. These often give the precise dates of marital quarrels, physical violence, previous suicide attempts, and other serious incidents.

In 1979 a woman accused of manslaughter had thirty previous convictions, occurring at cycles of 29.04 plus or minus 1.47 days (Figure 37; "fitted" cycles are those for which the precise dates of menstruation are only occasionally known, but there is accuracy regarding the events of violence or criminal acts). Also, numerous episode of bizarre behavior and violence occurred when she was in prison. Episodes of unruly behaviors were recorded by prison officers involved, and again her documents showed that while in prison she had made attempts at drowning and strangling herself, escaping, slashing her wrists, smashing windows, and setting fire to the bed in her cell. These incidents in prison were found to have occurred at intervals of 29.55 plus or minus 1.45 days (Figure 38).

Thus, the diagnosis did not rely on the woman's memory. Prison records also showed that she had been described as "pleasant and co-operative, but at times loses her senses and can be quite impulsive," which suggested that destructive symptoms were completely absent after menstruation.

An eighteen-year-old ballet dancer who was accused of arson successfully pleaded PMS as a mitigating factor and was released on probation. She had an excellent school record,

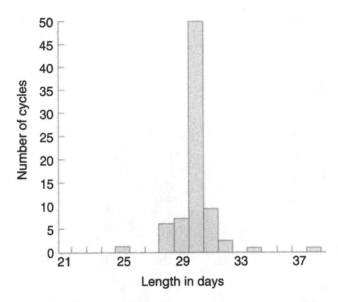

Figure 37 Distribution of "fitted" cycles between prison admissions

and her behavior had always been exemplary until she started menstruating. After that she appeared to change in character, and she had severe episodes of unusual and unexplained behavior. One day she suddenly went into her bedroom and shaved off her blonde hair and eyebrows; another time she ran away from home and was later returned by the police, having been found drunk and disorderly; once she burned the bedroom curtains; another time she overdosed on pain relievers and alcohol and was hospitalized for a night; finally, she set fire to her father's house and was sent to prison. While in prison, she tried to set fire to the bed in her cell. On another occasion, she attempted to strangle herself by tying one end of a sheet around her neck and the other end to the top of the window.

It was her father who noticed from his diaries that his daughter's problems occurred about once a month. He was advised to produce proof that would show the precise dates on which the different events occurred. He did this by searching through the doctor's and hospital's files, and by checking the dates of insurance claims for the burned curtains, the date on the

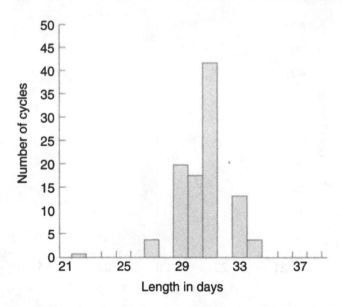

Figure 38 Distribution of "fitted" cycles between episodes of
               violence in prison

check with which he bought his daughter a new wig, and the precise dates on which she misbehaved while in prison. The many
incidents were clearly shown to have occurred in regular monthly
cycles. This was the first case in which PMS succeeded as a mitigating factor in arson. The girl received progesterone treatment
and is now a successful executive. (See *Nicola*, pages 253–254.)

A similar story is the one of an unemployed girl who
harassed the police with unnecessary emergency phone calls
(see *Anne*, pages 258–59). She had earlier been sent to a reform
school for the same offense, but after being released she persisted
with the calls and was imprisoned. Again, her father was the
one who noticed that the problems occurred every month and
told the lawyer. In her case the calls represented a cry for help,
akin to other women whose cry for attention might be a suicide
attempt or self-mutilation. She, too, responded to progesterone
and was released on probation. However, after she left prison
the progesterone was not continued, and she again began making unnecessary police phone calls. This time no mercy was

shown, and she served a two-year sentence. That was fifteen years ago; today, now that she is on progesterone treatment, her life has changed and she is working with people with disabilities, is happily married, and has one son.

In 1977 a forty-six-year-old part-time social worker was charged with shoplifting. In court she produced her diary, showing the days of confusion each month when she refused to leave the house. It showed that she had arranged her days at work accordingly. Her husband had recognized the cyclical symptoms and described how she would return from shopping with dog food, although they had no pets, or a child's ski outfit, although their own children were now grown. Together, the husband and wife had marked in the appointment book the days on which trouble might occur. All had been well until the social worker had agreed to alter her working days. The case was dismissed. She has since received progesterone treatment and has been free from these times of lapsed concentration and confusion.

These represent genuine cases of criminal behavior resulting from a hormonal disease that responds to treatment. These women deserve to be freed, for they cannot be held responsible for their unexpected loss of control. However, the genuine cases are few and far between, and it is important to ensure that PMS is not made a universal defense. Cases have already occurred in England where this has been tried. A woman on her first charge of shoplifting cannot claim PMS in her defense without evidence that this is a recurring problem The mere coincidence of two car crashes or two speeding offenses occurring in the premenstruum cannot be considered. If the woman recognizes she suffers from PMS, it is her responsibility to get treatment.

For a correct diagnosis, the precise dates of menstruation and of the alleged crime are necessary. Yet a clerk in a travel agency, accused of stealing traveler's checks worth $1,000 from her employee on some unknown date between August and April the following year, pleaded PMS. Not surprisingly, the plea failed and a jail sentence was imposed.

When a woman pleads PMS in her defense, the public still has a right to be protected by the knowledge that the defendant is receiving treatment and is unlikely to be a further danger. Because PMS is a recurrent illness, if the woman is not treated she is likely to repeat the offense, be it murder, assault, damage to property, or shoplifting. At an appeals trial in England, PMS was rejected as a defense in a case of murder, although it still stands as a "factor causing diminished responsibility" in capital charges, and "a mitigating factor" in lesser charges.

CHARACTERISTICS OF PMS OFFENSES

There are certain characteristics of the offenses committed by sufferers of PMS that may be easily recognized:

- The woman acts alone, without an accomplice.
- The offense is not premeditated, and it usually comes as a surprise even to those whom she was with shortly before the event.
- The action is without clear motive, such as setting fire to an unknown person's property.
- There may be no attempt to escape. A woman may randomly throw a brick in a shop window and then phone the police and await her arrest.
- The action may be a cri de coeur, as with the girl who repeatedly makes emergency 911 calls. This is similar to a suicide attempt.

Among the more frequent symptoms of PMS that may result in criminal acts is a sudden and momentary surge of uncontrollable emotion resulting in violence, confusion or amnesia, alcoholism, and attention-seeking episodes that represent cries for help. The resulting actions may cover a full range of criminal offenses such as actual violence, damage to property, theft, and disorderly behavior (see *Anna Reynolds, page 254*).

IDENTIFYING PMS OFFENDERS

Sufferers of PMS characteristically have pain-free menstruation (unless they have the additional diagnosis of pelvic inflammatory disease or endometriosis). The shoplifter who claimed her period pains were so severe that she was under the influence of pain-relieving drugs at the time of her offenses was suffering from spasmodic dysmenorrhea, not from PMS.

A full medical history will reveal information that can confirm or disprove the diagnosis. The onset of PMS and the occasions of increased severity always occur at times of hormonal upheaval, such as at puberty, during or after taking the Pill, or after amenorrhea, pregnancy, or sterilization. The women involved have side effects on the Pill, while preeclampsia or postnatal depression may complicate their pregnancy. During the premenstruum they have difficulty in tolerating long intervals without food (over five hours in the daytime or twelve hours overnight), and they become easily intoxicated by alcohol while in the premenstruum.

A thirty-two-year-old Essex housewife was accused of infanticide, having drowned her second daughter and then overdosed herself (see Jean, pages 259–260). She started menstruating in the intensive care unit, and mention of PMS was noted in her previous medical records. She had developed migraine and hypertension on the Pill, for which she was admitted for observation to the London Hospital. Her first pregnancy was complicated by preeclampsia, and after her second pregnancy she developed postnatal depression requiring psychiatric attention. The incident occurred about 5:30 P.M., and she had had no food since her 8:30 A.M. breakfast. The court accepted the several diagnostic pointers indicating PMS, and she was released on probation with the requirement that she receive treatment for PMS.

Among women with PMS, increased libido is occasionally noticed in the premenstruum, a fact recorded by Israel back in 1938. As mentioned before, this urge may be responsible for adolescent girls running away from home. These girls can be helped and their criminal career abruptly ended with hormone therapy.

The factors associated with sudden loss of control are shown in the box that follows.

Factors responsible for sudden loss of control

- Risk factors
  PMS stress
  Pill or progestogen
  Family history
  Smoker

- Immediate factors
  premenstruum
  long food gap
  sleep deficit, tired, late at night
  alcohol or drugs

Some women who suffer greatly from PMS are needlessly incarcerated. They are deserving of our sympathy, and justice will not be served until all true sufferers of PMS are properly diagnosed and treated. The road to rehabilitation after a prison sentence is long and hard.

The interests of all women will be served best by increasing our diagnostic capacity, enabling us to distinguish the few genuine PMS sufferers from the many malingerers whose claims of PMS can never be substantiated. Further information on this subject is contained in my book *Premenstrual Syndrome Goes to Court* (see "Other Publications by the Author," at end of book).

20

After a Hysterectomy or Oophorectomy

Many women who have endured menstrual miseries each month for years dream of the day when those troublesome organs will be removed by one stroke of the surgeon's knife. Can anyone blame them? Already, hysterectomy is such a common procedure that it is known as the Birthday Operation, to be celebrated in one's fortieth year, as this is the most common age for the operation in the United States. In the United States the phrase "total hysterectomy" is used to mean the removal of the womb, tubes, and ovaries, an operation known medically as HBSO, or hysterectomy with bilateral salpingo-oophorectomy. Medically, if the cervix is left after removal of the womb this is known as a subtotal hysterectomy. Only if the whole womb including the cervix is removed do surgeons call it a total hysterectomy. An oophorectomy is the removal of either one or both ovaries.

Today, the risks associated with the removal of the womb are minimal, and with the newer technique of keyhole surgery, or laparoscopical assisted vaginal hysterectomy (LAVH), postoperative pain and length of hospital stay are greatly reduced. But is it really the answer to a woman's prayers if the only reason is to end PMS? It is no good asking the gynecologist, who sees the woman a few weeks later, examines the scar to see if it has healed well, assures her that she will never menstruate again, possibly prescribes some estrogen tablets, and says good-bye. It is better to ask the family physician, who will care for this woman not just for one year but for the next twenty years, or you can ask the woman herself.

There are many very good reasons for removing the womb, and possibly the ovaries as well. At the top of the list comes the possibility of any malignancy. Sometimes it is done because of fibroids, when they are either so large that they interfere with another organ or so numerous that they cause heavy menstruation resulting in anemia. Another good reason is because of endometriosis. There are also women who do it so as to be 100 percent contraceptively safe, who do not want the problems associated with the Pill and other methods of contraception, possibly because they have already tried those methods without success. A forty-two-year-old boutique owner confided to me that she had changed her gynecologist seven times before she found one who was prepared to remove her womb for contraception. She just did not feel convinced that sterilization would be reliable enough.

If a hysterectomy is needed, then the removal of the ovaries also needs to be considered. Facts in favor of their removal are the ever-present possibility of ovarian cancer developing and the knowledge that in premenopausal women ovaries tend to decrease in activity within two or three years of hysterectomy. The women can then receive hormone replacement, but that is only an argument if the individual is known to respond to estrogen. Far too many women have a hysterectomy in order to overcome their PMS. There are gynecologists who argue that if one removes menstruation, the premenstruum does not exist and so PMS can no longer occur. That is correct, but these women still suffer cyclical recur-rences of the symptoms of the syndrome at the times of their missed menstruation, usually known as post-hysterectomy syn-drome, or PHS. The operation is in the pelvis, not in the brain, where the menstrual control center is situated, and the stimulating hormones from the menstrual center continue to be released in their usual monthly pattern. Observations of symptoms kept on menstrual charts by women who have had a hysterectomy clearly show a menstrual pattern. Indeed, study of such charts also shows which women had long cycles of thirty-two days compared to those who habitually had short cycles, nearer three weeks (see Figure 39).

There are other gynecologists who wrongly state that PMS does not occur in anovular cycles, so they recommend treatment of PMS by suppression of ovulation, which can be achieved by

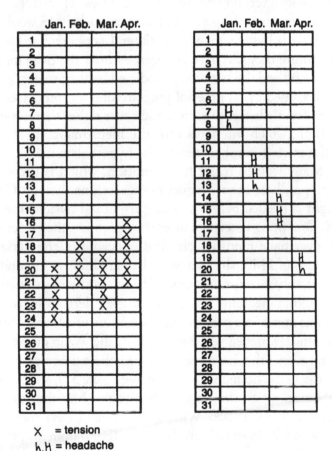

X   = tension

h, H = headache

Figure 39   Menstrual charts of post-hysterectomy syndrome

the Pill, estrogen, or danol (gonadotrophin release inhibitor). The Pill increases PMS, so that is a nonstarter. If estrogen is given continuously, it may cause a buildup of the lining of the womb, with pathological changes and possibly cancer. Therefore, with estrogen therapy there must be regular shedding of the womb lining with bleeding, which is achieved by giving progestogen at the end of each monthly course of estrogen. As would be expected, the progestogens cause PMS-like symptoms, which can be every bit as bad as the PMS that the treatment is designed to relieve! In fact, John Studd, a London gynecologist, states that after having received courses of estrogen and progestogen, some 10 percent of women with PMS would prefer to have a hysterectomy and bilateral oophorectomy so that in the future they can have estrogen without the need for regular bleeding and the symptoms produced by the progestogens. If PMS is caused by an upset of progesterone receptors (see page 91), it is surely better to correct the cause rather than submit to castration, which interferes with the menstrual control center and the other control centers in the hypothalamus.

Many women regret the operation, which is irrevocable and may still require subsequent progesterone therapy. Careful thought is needed before agreeing to a total hysterectomy for PMS. One thing is certain: after the operation the patient will no longer have monthly bleeding. Because of the variety of symptoms of PMS, she may later be cared for by the endocrinologist, psychiatrist, rheumatologist, cardiologist, neurologist, internal medicine physician, or even dermatologist.

The immediate postoperative weeks are usually pleasant and uneventful. However, whether it is only the womb or the womb and the ovaries that have been removed, there is now an irreparable break in the hormonal pathway (see Figure 37), and the menstrual clock, which the surgeon did not touch in the operation, receives a severe shock. Within six to eight days there is an increase in follicle-stimulating hormone (FSH) from the pituitary, and within eight to ten days an increase in luteinizing hormone (LH). The menstrual clock then reacts to the lack of information from the womb, and over the next three weeks there is a threefold increase in FSH, while the amount of LH doubles and continues at the abnormally high level for years. This increase is not as great if an estrogen implant is inserted at the time of operation.

ARTIFICIAL MENOPAUSE

The changes that accompany the surgical removal of the womb or ovaries are known as "artificial menopause" and should not be confused with natural menopause. The changes in natural menopause occur gradually over an average of five years, as the menstrual clock slowly closes down and the ovaries and womb shrink. In artificial menopause the changes are sudden and affect only the womb and/or the ovaries, leaving intact the menstrual clock, which continues its menstrual cycle until the time of natural menopause.

All goes well for about six to twelve months after the operation, whether the woman is having HRT or not, but once the initial trauma of the operation is over and the menstrual control center is healed, the hormonal differences between the two groups of women shown in Figures 41 and 42. Those who previously suffered from PMS will find that their cyclical symptoms return. The husband may be the first to notice and say something. Or the woman may recognize the telltale headache that previously ushered in a period, and which now assumes the proportions of a devastating migraine.

Angela, the forty-eight-year-old wife of a USAF colonel, had a successful hysterectomy for fibroids that had been causing heavy bleeding (see page 260). She had an excellent recovery, until nine months later, when she suddenly had four days of extreme tiredness. She stayed in bed, blaming it on a virus. The following month it happened again, and this time she stayed in bed for six days. Gradually, the duration of the tiredness increased, until it took two weeks out of every month. It would start gradually, as a general tiredness, and she would manage to keep going for a few days, but soon, bed rest became essential.

The end of each attack was quite definite, and afterward she was free of symptoms and could resume her normal social life.

Her husband had kept a meticulous diary, from which a chart was made. She had already had nine months of this distressing condition when I first saw her. Fortunately, it responded completely to progesterone treatment.

Premenstrual syndrome always increases in severity after a hysterectomy, and there may also be extra symptoms. One woman, a part-time worker, was sent to me after she had been charged with shoplifting. Two years previously she had had a hysterectomy, and prior to the operation she had suffered from premenstrual tension and headaches. After the operation her PMS became worse, and for a few days of each month she would also experience breast fullness and feelings of unreality and confusion. She carefully charted these days on a calendar and related the episodes to the times of her expected premenstruum. She then arranged her work schedule to avoid stress on these days of inevitable confusion. In court she described the nature of the confusion, how sometimes she would come home having bought items she did not need, such as dog food, though she had no dogs, highly spiced foods that she never ate, and underwear that was the wrong size. She would be in a daze and could not tell what was happening. The day of her offense had been such a day. After she had been charged, when she was being taken to the police station by a plainclothes policeman, she thought the officer was a rapist who was driving her down an unknown road. The case was dismissed. She has since undergone progesterone treatment and is now free from cyclical confusion and PMS.

In 1975, during a British nationwide survey of the hormonal factors affecting migraines in women, it was noted that women with a history of PMS said that the severity of their migraines had been increased by a hysterectomy. Their three-month charts, giving the precise timing of migraine attacks, confirmed that the attacks were still occurring cyclically.

The need for women with cyclical symptoms to keep careful records and charts of their problems, even if they have had their womb or ovaries removed, cannot be emphasized too strongly. If it is difficult to record days of depression because the onset is gradual, it may be just as useful to record the days on which breast symptoms occur, as these usually start more suddenly. Alternatively, really good days may be recorded with a simple check mark.

Brenda, forty-seven years old, began her consultation with a detailed account of how her husband had been moved from one town to another, and how she had made a suicide attempt within days of their move and had been hospitalized for several months. Within a week or two of her discharge, she moved back to her previous home, but she made another suicide attempt the following week and was once again hospitalized. Only after giving a long and confused history, assisted by her husband, did she mention that she had had a hysterectomy and was now experiencing cyclical attacks of depression and moodiness. Once the cyclical nature of her symptoms was confirmed by a two-month record, she was given progesterone treatment, which helped restore normalcy.

Two surveys done in 1975 indicated a high incidence of depression in women one to three years after a hysterectomy, with or without the removal of the ovaries. The depression appears to be greatest in those who were under forty years old at the time of the operation; those with a previous history of depression, especially postnatal depression; those in whom no gynecological abnormality could be found by the pathologist who examined the womb after operation (in one of the surveys, 45 percent of the wombs were reported to be normal); and those who had a history of marital problems.

Dr. Ronald Richards, a general practitioner in Oxford, England, observed that patients who had undergone hysterectomies often had medical notes bulging out of their files, so that one could tell at a glance that they had already been in and out of many hospital departments. His survey, confirmed by others, emphasized the high incidence of depression in those with a history of hysterectomy.

My paper "The Aftermath of Hysterectomy and Oophorectomy," read at the Royal Society of Medicine in London in 1957, revealed that 44 percent of women had either been divorced, separated, or seen a marriage counselor since the operation. One reason could be lack of understanding or empathy on the part of husbands, who believe that the cause of the menstrual problems has been removed. The comments of two husbands were as follows:

> She used to have a reason for it, but now she's quite unpredictable.

> I thought the operation would make her more even-tempered.

Another disturbing finding in the survey was that over 50 percent of the women gained more than twenty-eight pounds in the year following their hysterectomy. How often is a woman warned before the operation that the odds are two to one that such a marked weight gain will occur? The reason for the depression and weight gain after hysterectomy may be related to the proximity of the menstrual clock to the mood-controlling and weight-controlling centers in the hypothalamus (see Figure 40).

There seem to be two types of post-hysterectomy depression: a cyclical depression and a continuous depression. The continuous depression is more likely to affect those who experienced spasmodic dysmenorrhea in their youth and have a tendency to be estrogen-deficient. These women respond very well to estrogen therapy, which needs to be continued through their depressive illness and well after the time of the natural menopause. The estrogen is given continually, as there is no risk of it causing a buildup of the lining of the womb. If the depression is cyclical, it will respond to progesterone. This should also be given continually, even if ovulation is still occurring, as there is no longer the possibility of causing irregularity of menstruation.

If only a hysterectomy has been performed, ovulation will continue, but with the interruption of the hormonal pathway

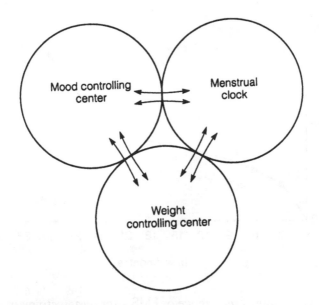

Figure 40   Diagram of controlling centers in the hypothalamus

there may be a gradual deterioration of ovarian function and a premature menopause. In these cases, as well as in the case of women who have had both ovaries removed, there is a decrease in bone mineral density and a risk of developing osteoporosis. These women need hormone replacement therapy; they will also benefit from moderate daily exercise and should appreciate the importance of calcium and vitamin D in their diet.

A few women develop a high prolactin level, suggesting that the operation has caused a disturbance in the hypothalamic-pituitary mechanism. They usually respond well to bromocriptine, a drug that lowers the prolactin level.

In theory, the removal of the womb should have no effect on sexual activity. The vagina and clitoris are untouched and, if anything, sexual activity should be enhanced once the fear of becoming pregnant is permanently removed. In practice, however, some women who previously had a satisfactory sex life suddenly find that they have lost their sexual zest and enjoyment. If this happens it is worth seeking professional help; often, testosterone can be a magic restorative.

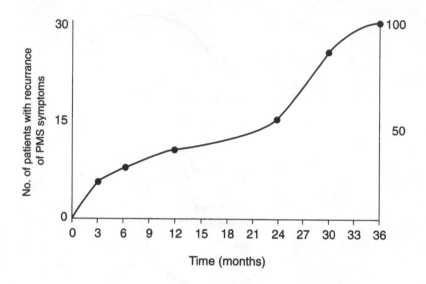

Figure 41   Time of recurrence of PMS after hysterectomy in
thirty women

Recently I analyzed current files and retrieved files of
eighty-nine women who had previously had a hysterectomy,
including fifty-one who had the operation solely because of
PMS. Among these fifty-one women 58 percent had a recurrence within six months and 98 percent within three years; it
was the women who had had their ovaries removed whose
PMS symptoms returned earliest (Figures 41 and 42).

The two previous studies on the relief of PMS following
hysterectomy by Casson and his team and by Casper and his
team, both in 1990, were followed up for only eight months
after the operations. My study is the first study of a cohort of
post-hysterectomy PMS patients that has been followed up for
as long as three years. The disturbing feature of my study was
that the women had normal wombs and ovaries removed, hoping for symptomatic relief, and then found they were unable to
tolerate estrogen replacement therapy. There was a difference
both before and after the operation of the inability of the

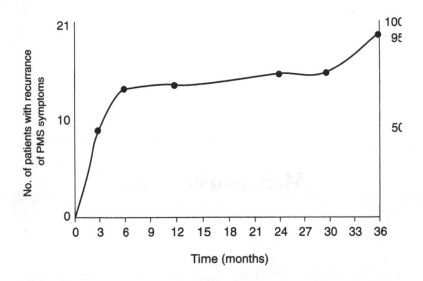

Figure 42 Time of recurrence of PMS after hysterectomy and
bilateral oophorectomy

group to tolerate estrogen or progestogen, and in the benefit
they received from progesterone therapy.

Research has shown that when female apes have their
wombs removed, their partner rejects them. But if the ape is
only given a mock operation and the womb is not removed,
the apes enjoy a natural sexual relationship. Whether a similar effect occurs in humans is not known, because we do not
carry out mock operations on humans.

21

*

Menopausal Years

It is only children who long to grow old—adults hate the very thought of it. This is especially true for women when menopause approaches. Many women see this as a doorway leading to old age and senility—when it is really the gateway to an era of serenity, a time characterized by confidence, calmness, sophistication, stable moods, and endless energy. In previous editions this chapter was called "Menopausal Miseries," but I have changed the title because miseries need no longer be anticipated or be present during these years of reproductive change. The physiological changes of puberty prepare the female for the era of childbearing. While occasionally these years may be tempestuous and one does meet some awkward adolescents, in fact, most girls pass through these changes without any major troubles. Menopause is the opposite of puberty. It is when the physiological changes are preparing the female for the era when childbearing is over; and while some may have problems during the changeover, the majority will pass through these years without any major troubles.

Women are unique in the animal kingdom as the only females who outlive their reproductive function and can then enjoy up to half their life span without it. Their menstrual clock runs at its own individual rate, and the end of menstruation occurs according to an individual, prearranged plan. In some the clock runs on a little longer, while in others it stops earlier.

The word *menopause* means the pausing of menstruation, and more precisely, the last menstruation. It cannot be timed as accurately as the menarche because it is seen only in retrospect; only when there have been no menstruations for a year can it be dated exactly. Earlier, the term *climacteric* was used to cover the years before and after the last menstruation, a time when changes were occurring in the reproductive system. Nowadays it is usual to use the term *menopause* more loosely to cover all the years of hormonal change.

HORMONAL CHANGES

As with all the changes Nature makes in our reproductive system, those at menopause are very gradual, taking between five and seven years to complete. First, there is the occasional missed ovulation. Studies have shown that the occasional anovular cycle can occur up to six years before the last menstruation. Gradually, missed ovulations become more frequent, and the menstrual flow becomes lighter and scantier. As the ovaries decline, the hypothalamus and pituitary try to stimulate them with an increased output of follicle-stimulating hormone (FSH) and luteinizing hormone (LH). But the ovaries are unable to respond; their production of estrogen and progesterone gradually decreases and over a few years stops entirely (see Figure 43). Thus, the presence of menopause can be determined by blood tests showing a low level of estradiol and a raised level of FSH.

Just as we now know that a small amount of progesterone is necessary for both sexes throughout life, there is also a small amount of estrogen present throughout life in both sexes. During the menstrual years, the main functions of estrogen are rebuilding the lining of the womb after it has been shed at menstruation, altering the cervical mucus to assist fertilization,

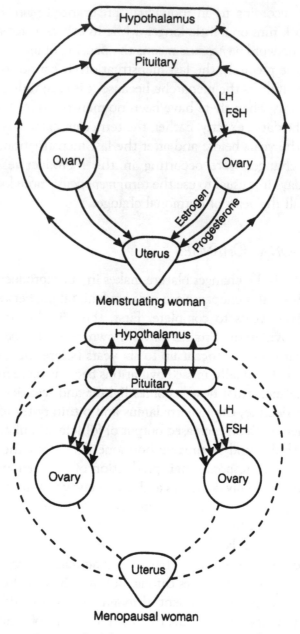

Figure 43   Hormonal pathways in menstruating and menopausal women

and breast development. It also has other functions that are especially important when the menstruating years are over. Estrogen promotes cholesterol balance, nourishes the circulatory system, increases the elasticity of the skin, and is involved in building up the bones. Throughout life, in both men and women, the two adrenal glands build up progesterone from cholesterol and then convert it further into estrogen, testosterone, cortisone, and other steroids. When estrogen is no longer produced by the ovaries, a menopausal estrogen called estrone is produced in the adrenal glands and in the peripheral tissues. After menopause it is this nonovarian estrogen, estrone, that has to fulfill the other functions for the blood, bones, and skin. Often, there is insufficient estrogen for these other tasks—either temporarily, during the changeover time, or permanently—and it is this lack of estrogen that is responsible for many of the unpleasant symptoms of menopause. Then the woman, once her ovaries decline, may be left to carry on without a sufficiency of this vital and powerful female hormone.

Up to the age of forty, narrowing of the arteries—particularly of the blood vessels of the heart—and coronary thrombosis are between ten and forty times more common in men than in women. After menopause, as the circulating estrogen decreases, there is a marked increase in narrowing of the arteries in women, so that gradually the difference between men and women decreases. But it is not until the age of seventy-five that the incidence is equal. It has been suggested that this may be due to insufficient progesterone, for it has now been appreciated that progesterone receptors are in the innermost lining cells of the blood vessels (endothelial cells). After the sudden menopause that occurs following a hysterectomy, the incidence of narrowing of the arteries and coronary vessels is increased four times as compared with premenopausal women. Also, among the few women who have a premature menopause before the age of forty, there is a sevenfold increase in coronary thrombosis. So the presence of estrogen in the blood is very important in preventing narrowing of the arteries and the occurrence of coronary disease.

Bones are not stable, unchanging structures. Throughout life, new bone cells are being laid down and old ones removed. This requires calcium, phosphorus, vitamins, and other minerals, as well as estrogen and progesterone. This is why everyone—men, women, and children included—has a small amount of estrogen and progesterone circulating in their blood. This estrogen is produced by the two adrenal glands. After menopause, those women whose bodies have relied during their menstruating life on the estrogen produced by the ovaries may find they have insufficient estrogen being made by the adrenals. This leads to thinning of the bones. This loss of bone mass shows up on special scans that estimate bone mineral density. This test is usually carried out on the lumbar vertebrae, the neck of the femur, or the ulnar bone of the wrist. Ten years after menopause a decrease in bone density is present in 40 percent of all women. The test can foretell if an individual is a possible candidate for osteoporosis in the future twenty years. Those at risk of osteoporosis, or brittle bone disease, can be treated with hormone replacement, either estrogen or progesterone. If osteoporosis is already present there is now treatment to build up the bones, with either etidronate or alendronate. It is a slow process, so the earlier treatment is started, the better. It is advised that all women at fifty should have a bone mineral density test, to ensure that there will be adequate time to treat those at risk.

Studies are showing that many factors are involved in causing osteoporosis. These include episodes of amenorrhea or anovulation and excessive athletic training during the menstruating years; bilateral tubal ligation before the age of thirty-five; and treatment with steroids, thyroxine, diuretics, and insulin. There is also a marked family incidence.

After menstruation ceases, progesterone is no longer required to prepare the lining of the womb or the cervical mucus for possible pregnancy, but progesterone also has another function. All through life, in both sexes, progesterone is built up in the adrenal glands from cholesterol and immediately converted into estrogen, testosterone, and the stress hormones, cortisone and corticosteroids. As ovarian progesterone is present in the bloodstream for only half of each cycle, the adrenals generally manage to make enough for their own needs during the menstruating years, and so they are usually capable of carrying on this task after menopause. This is why progesterone deficiency is no longer such a problem after menopause, although if progesterone is given it can be converted into estrogen.

TWO HORMONAL GROUPS

Women can be divided into two hormonal types: the estrogen-responsive and the progesterone-responsive. Most of this book has dealt with the progesterone-responsive group and the problems that can be caused by PMS in the home, at work, and at play. At menopause we return to the estrogen-responsive group, for these are the women whose menopausal sufferings begin earliest and are the most severe. This is illustrated in Figure 44, which shows that women who had spasmodic dysmenorrhea in their teens and then sufficient estrogen for normal menstruation nevertheless suffer most from menopausal symptoms. In fact, the chances are that they will begin to experience menopausal symptoms while still menstruating regularly each month. They really need estrogen therapy at the menopause, and probably for many years thereafter. Women who were in the normal category may require estrogen therapy during the changeover period but will probably manage to make enough for their own requirements thereafter. Women who suffered from mild PMS may require estrogen temporarily when their menstruation first stops, but gradually they usually find they can manage without it. The severe PMS sufferers will probably have no need for estrogen, either during the menopausal years or later; they always have a high estrogen level, with ovarian estrogen supplemented by that produced in the adrenals. But they will benefit from progesterone, probably for many years.

In short, it is what we call in England a case of roundabouts and swings. Those who had greatest difficulties with

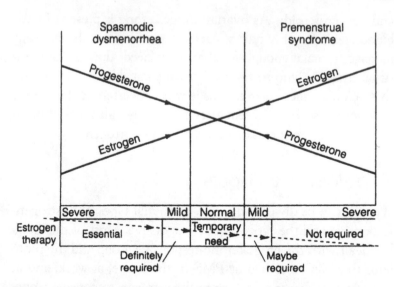

Figure 44   Need for estrogen therapy at menopause

premenstrual monthly problems can now look forward to a problem-free era, while those who had little trouble during their twenties and thirties will probably face the most problems at menopause.

Throughout this book I have avoided using the term *hormone replacement therapy*, or HRT, to avoid confusion. Both estrogen and progesterone are hormones, and both are used in replacement therapy. In the mind of the public and the media, HRT has become limited to the use of estrogen plus progestogen therapy during menopause, while the letters ERT are used to denote estrogen replacement therapy. The term *hormone replacement therapy* has also been used for years by doctors when giving insulin to diabetics and thyroxine to those with hypothyroid disease.

AGE OF MENOPAUSE

In the United States the average age of menopause is fifty-two, while in Britain it is fifty, with a range of forty-five to fifty-five. Those whose menstruation ceases before they are forty-five years old are said to have a "premature menopause."

The exact age of menopause is very individual. However, four factors can give some indication of whether it is likely to be early or late:

- The age of menarche. Those who start menstruation early tend to finish late, so there is a "rainbow" effect, as shown in Figure 45.
- The hormonal group. Those in the estrogen-responsive group have a tendency to finish menstruation early, while sufferers from PMS tend to finish after they are fifty.
- Genetic factors. If your mother, sisters, and aunts finished menstruation early, you may also expect to finish early. For this reason it is worth finding out at what age your mother had her last normal menstruation. If she had an easy change of life, the chances are that you, too, will have an easy time. If your mother suffered, make sure you receive the benefits of modern medicine.
- Smoking. A survey at a medical center in London showed that at forty-eight to forty-nine years, 36 percent of smokers were postmenopausal compared with 23 percent nonsmokers; four years later, the figures were 89 percent for smokers and 71 percent for nonsmokers. So smoking habits should also be considered when estimating the probable age at which menopause may occur.

PATTERNS OF ENDING

The charts of women who regularly record the dates of their menstruation show that the menstruating years end in a wide variety of ways. Three patterns are recognizable, but some women will find that their own individual ending covers more than one pattern:

1. There is a gradual ending. Where menstruation initially lasted four or five days, it gradually lasts one or two days, then only one day or even one hour monthly. Generally, the cycle is maintained and menstruation comes when expected.

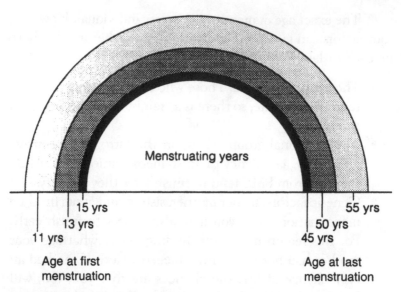

Figure 45 Relation between age of menarche and menopause

2. There is an occasional missed menstruation, possibly just one, and then menstruation resumes again for two or three months before another is missed. Gradually, there are more missed menstruations than actual menstruations, but each menstruation lasts the expected number of days, for example, four to six days.

3. There is a sudden ending of menstruation, which had previously been regular, with the final menstruation lasting the normal or nearly normal number of days. This abrupt ending is most likely to coincide with a stressful event, such as a daughter's wedding, moving, or becoming a grandparent. This abrupt ending may even be the start of a depressive illness, and it is usually accompanied by the fear of pregnancy.

The effect of the first missed or delayed menstruation often depends on the woman's recent sexual activity and desire for pregnancy. If she has not been sexually active, she may not notice the infrequency or absence of menstrual bleeding for a month or more. If she has been sexually active, she may become concerned and increasingly happy or unhappy with each additional day of missed menstruation. While the possibility of pregnancy is usually uppermost in the minds of women whose regular menstruation suddenly stops, after a woman is forty-five she should always consider the possibility that menopause has begun. Comments by alarmed patients in this predicament include these:

I don't want to get my name in the Guinness Book of Records as the oldest mother in the world.

I would hate to be drawing my old age pension when my child is at school.

And from a grandmother:

My child would be younger than her niece.

It is usually quite easy for a doctor to tell if a patient is pregnant or is starting menopause. Today a simple blood or urine test will settle the question of whether or not missed menstruation is due to early pregnancy. Before such technology was available, a doctor's examination would settle the question. If she was pregnant, her breasts would be full, she might have symptoms of morning sickness and of passing urine during the night, and on examination her vagina would be red and moist and the neck of the womb soft. On the other hand, if she was entering her menopause, her breasts would begin to decrease in size and firmness, she might experience menopausal symptoms, especially hot flashes, and on examination her vagina would be pale and dry and the neck of the womb firm and smaller. The most characteristic symptom of menopause is the hot flush or hot flash. It is a sensation of burning heat, arising from the waist and passing up to the top of the head. It lasts only a few minutes, five at the most, and may either be visible, when the skin becomes flushed and beads of sweat appear, or invisible.

Very few women indeed pass through their menopausal years without experiencing a single flash, which may range in frequency from only one or two a week to between fifty and one hundred a day. They embarrass many women, but others working with women of their own age can laugh about them, believing that "a flash shared is a flash halved." Our grandparents used to say they were worth "a dollar a flash." Hot flashes may be accompanied by palpitations, a fluttering in the chest, or a feeling of choking, apprehension, or anxiety, and they are worse immediately after a hot drink or spicy food and if there has been a long interval between food. If the hot flashes last longer than half an hour, then there is likely to be some other cause for them. The flashes can occur at night, when the woman may awaken abruptly in a bath of sweat. These are known as night sweats.

There is a story about a group of women undergraduates at Girton College, Cambridge, in the 1920s, who were discussing the menopausal problems and hot flashes that their mothers and counselors were experiencing. They agreed that because they were all emancipated and fully understood the facts of life, they would never have to suffer the same ordeals. They formed a Menopause Club, promising to keep in touch with each other and exchange full accounts of how they fared through that great age. When the time came, each one of them experienced the flashes and other menopausal symptoms to a greater or lesser degree, despite their full knowledge of the events of life. The flashes are thought to be caused by a sudden stimulus to the temperature-controlling center in the hypothalamus and are associated with a rise in FSH and LH from the pituitary, as well as a deficiency of estrogen. Thus they are hormonal and not psychological.

MENOPAUSAL SYMPTOMS

Menopausal symptoms are usually divided into two groups: specific symptoms, which are caused by estrogen deficiency and can be relieved by giving estrogen, and nonspecific psychological symptoms, some of which may be relieved by estrogen and some not, depending on the individual patient. These are illustrated in Figure 46.

Nonspecific symptoms include tiredness, insomnia, irritability, depression, headaches, palpitations, anxiety, dizziness, forgetfulness, and absentmindedness. The psychological symptoms may be secondary results of the primary symptoms, a so-called domino effect. Thus, the flashes, sweats, painful intercourse, and need to urinate frequently at night may cause insomnia and in turn lead to tiredness, irritability, and depression.

Hot flashes and sweats are usually the first signs of estrogen deficiency. Lack of estrogen may cause the vagina to become dry, pale, thin, and less resilient. There is a change in the acidity of the vagina, which leads to a change in the bacteria found there and a tendency to atrophic vaginitis and to infection. This in turn may cause itching, pain, or frequency in passing urine, especially at night (often misdiagnosed as cystitis). There is pain on initial penetration at intercourse and, ultimately, loss of sex drive.

The skin becomes paler and thinner and loses its elasticity, so that wrinkles develop, especially on the face around the eyes and mouth and on the neck. The soaring sales of cosmetics and beauty treatments and the demand for cosmetic surgery are evidence of the obvious distress caused by these symptoms of middle age.

The rheumatic-like pains that develop in the bones, muscles, and joints are due to the thinning of the bones. There is often considerable stiffness in the morning, and the pains tend to move around from one place to another over time. Sometimes the joints of the fingers become very painful and swollen, and as the pain and swelling decrease, the joints may be left deformed and misaligned. These vague, generalized joint pains may be early signs of loss of bone mass, or osteoporosis (see page 196), and are a warning that in the postmenopausal years, fractures of the wrist and the neck of the

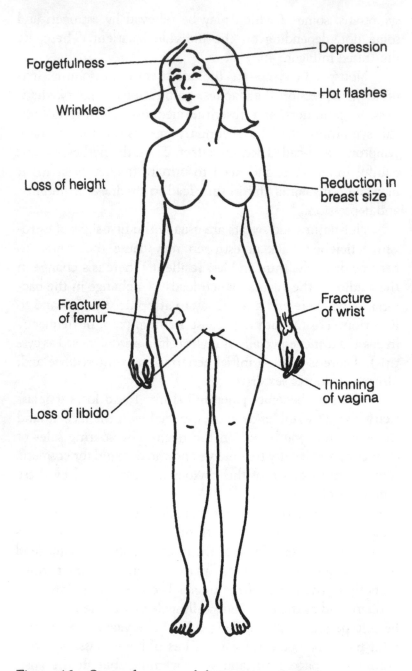

Figure 46 Signs of estrogen deficiency at menopause

femur and crushed fractures of the spine are likely to occur. The typical "dowager's hump" at the top of the spine is also a sign of thinning of the bones, but this generally does not develop until a woman is in her seventies.

Osteoporosis also causes a decrease in body height. Leonardo da Vinci, in his *Universal Man*, showed that in humans the height equals the armspan. This is true for men and premenopausal women. As a woman's vertebrae become thinner after menopause, however, there is a decrease in height, with no corresponding decrease in armspan. If the difference between the armspan and height exceeds an inch and a half, it is an indication that the woman should receive long-term hormone therapy (see Figure 47).

The greatest bone loss occurs early in menopause when menstruation is altering and becoming irregular, and for about two years after the last menstruation. Then the bone loss slowly reduces over the next twenty years. Gradually, the changes may lead to what has been called "little old lady" syndrome: "little" because height is lost, fat is reduced, and possibly there is spinal curvature; "old" because this happens after menopause; and "lady" because the development of osteoporosis is about five times more common in women than in men. All this results from the loss of estrogen, for the estrogen receptors in the bones still require the hormone, but there is much that can be done to prevent it (see chapter 22).

The worst symptoms are the nonspecific ones, which can lead to comments like these:

I think I must be going insane.

I feel so harassed; the whole world seems to be resting on my shoulders.

It's even tougher than pregnancy and labor.

The mood changes at menopause are continuous, not like premenstrual mood swings that last about two weeks and are

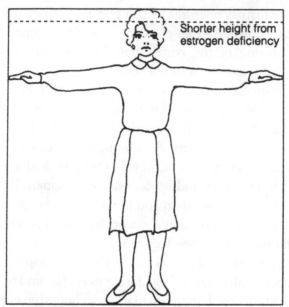

Normally the armspan equals the height, but if estrogen deficiency occurs at menopause the armspan exceeds the height

Figure 47 Relation between armspan and height

then eased, at least temporarily. They can turn an easygoing woman into a nag, a high-strung person into a crying hysteric, a happy-go-lucky individual into a restless bundle of nerves, and an efficient housewife into an absentminded professor type, who puts the cat in the refrigerator and the milk out the door. Many women choose this time to leave the femininity rat race, and their personality factors become more important—and possibly exaggerated. The woman's shape alters as her breasts begin to sag, and she develops middle-aged spread. There is a tendency for the thin to become even thinner and the fat to become obese.

DIAGNOSIS

It is essential to differentiate the diagnosis of menopause symptoms from those due to PMS. PMS may be present mildly for years, and them become severe in the forties. Fortunately, as mentioned earlier, menopause can be positively diagnosed by estimation of the FSH in a single blood test. If the FSH level is raised, ovulation is no longer occurring and the patient is in menopause.

MENOPAUSE
can be diagnosed by
RAISED FSH LEVEL

PMS sufferers also go through menopause as their menstruating years end, and if they continue with their usual regime of the Three-Hourly Starch Diet and progesterone they will hardly notice it and may well be completely free from symptoms. The treatment of the two conditions, PMS and menopause, are quite different; giving estrogen with progestogen to sufferers of PMS will only increase PMS, because the progestogens lower the blood progesterone level (see page 74). For this reason, a clear diagnosis of PMS or menopause is needed.

Menopause is usually not difficult to diagnose clinically. The hot flashes are the most obvious characteristic, but it must be remembered that hot flashes can also result from other conditions, such as when taking antidepressants or experiencing a drop in the blood sugar level. Thin skin, graying hair, wrinkles, vaginal dryness, and deformed fingers and toes are all obvious signs of menopause. If the bones are badly affected, there will also be a rise in blood calcium and phosphates. There used to be a simple test that doctors would perform to examine some vaginal cells under a microscope. Cells with ample estrogen have a dark, well-marked nucleus. This is known as the Karyopicnotic Index (or K.I.) test, and it is often done routinely when a cervical smear is performed, but an FSH estimation is more reliable.

If the diagnosis of menopause is in doubt, the woman may be given a month's trial of estrogen. If she reports an improvement, the prescription can be repeated. While there is frequently a beneficial placebo effect from giving tablets, if the benefit is maintained over two or three months, it strongly suggests that the hormone treatment is doing good.

The effect of menopause on sexual activity depends on a woman's experience during her menstruating years. If sex was important, then it is likely to be even more enjoyable once the fear of pregnancy is removed. If there never was much sexual excitement, then many think of menopause as a time when sexual activity may be slowed down or stopped. If estrogen is deficient, causing vaginal soreness and pain at penetration, the pain can be relieved by giving estrogen, either in the form of a cream applied locally or as tablets.

Some who talk and write—in error—about the "male menopause" describe it as a time when a man's sexual urge diminishes. This seems to be a kind of reverse chauvinism, which is doubly regrettable because it gives the impression that this is what is happening to women at menopause, which is quite wrong.

When Neuergarten was carrying out his study on attitudes toward menopause, he asked the loaded question, "What is the best thing about menopause?" Forty-four percent replied "not having to bother about menstruation," 30 percent said, "not being worried about getting pregnant," and 14 percent said "a better relationship with my husband and greater enjoyment of sex life."

In 1969, the International Health Foundation studied the subject and interviewed two thousand women who were between the ages of forty-five and fifty-five. Seventy-two percent agreed that after menopause it was good to be free from menstruation. Figures for the various countries ranged from 66 percent in Italy to 79 percent in the United Kingdom. It is tragic that since 1969 the media and the multinational pharmaceuticals have painted the menopausal years as a difficult and unpleasant time, a time that will require the help of hormones to ease the miseries, because this is not usually nor necessarily the case.

EMPTY NEST SYNDROME

Unfortunately, the menopausal years are often traumatic for women in other ways. It has been calculated that in the space of five years around her fiftieth birthday, the average woman will lose her mother through death, lose her daughter through marriage, and become a grandparent. There are also those homemakers whose children leave home for college or other employment, or who move because their husband makes a last career change or receives his final promotion. This has led psychologists to believe that all the miseries of menopause are just a woman's reaction to these losses—the so-called Empty Nest Syndrome. While many women are upset by these events, and their turmoil may cause emotional impulses to reach the menstrual clock in the hypothalamus, in the majority of cases if menopausal symptoms are present, they have a hormonal basis and respond well to hormone therapy.

With all the talk of the menopause, it is too easy for both doctors and patients to think that all symptoms experienced for the first time between the ages of forty-five and fifty-five are due to the physiological changes of menopause, and therefore to ignore the possibility of another diagnosis. There are so many other diseases that commonly start during these years that a full examination is recommended before automatically starting on hormone replacement. Some diseases, which creep up gradually and then become severe enough to need medical help, include raised blood pressure, thyroid disease, diabetes, and rheumatoid arthritis. All can be easily diagnosed with a few simple tests. Remember that it is always possible to have a double diagnosis, the menopause and some other illness, both of which need attention and treatment.

22

— ❧ —

Approach to Treatment

A disease with no universally recognized cause is always sub-ject to numerous suggested treatments. Some have never been tested, others result from old wives' tales, and many rely on the treatment of the main symptom. But PMS usually presents many symptoms, both psychological and physical, in the same patient. If one accepts the advanced medical knowledge that progesterone receptors are at the root of the problems of PMS, then the treatment approach should be aimed at relieving all the many symptoms, psychological and physical, of PMS by ensuring maximum functioning of progesterone receptors. This entails:

- Consideration of the current lifestyle.
- Relief of stress (see chapter 23).
- Maintenance of a stable blood sugar level (see Three-Hourly Starch Diet, chapter 24).
- Progesterone replacement therapy (see chapter 25).

However, if there is only one PMS symptom, such as asthma, which can be controlled well with bronchodilators and inhalers, then it is best to ease the PMS symptoms with con-ventional treatment, and at the same time change to the Three-Hourly Starch Diet (see page 223). Whether the diagnosis of

PMS is possible, probable, or positive, it is easy enough to correct the diet, while trying to improve the lifestyle.

PRELIMINARIES

The therapist will need to take a full medical and social history, which should include the ability to tolerate the Pill and any previous preeclampsia or postnatal depression, as a higher dose of progesterone is likely to be needed later.

The patient needs to be instructed in the use of the menstrual chart, which she may have prepared in advance, or she may be able to fill it up from the appointment book she keeps in her handbag. As a diagnosis of PMS depends solely on the timing of symptoms in relation to menstruation, it is essential to record full details of *exact* dates of symptoms and menstruation. There is no place for guess dates or vague dates thought up at the spur of the moment at the consultation. It is recommended to chart only the three most severe symptoms; nevertheless, the therapist should make notes of all other symptoms mentioned at the first consultation.

It is wise to have written knowledge of the patient's normal diet, on both weekdays and weekends, before attempting to discuss the Three-Hourly Starch Diet. In an active daily life, most of us have faults in our diet, and often it is only when we have actually written down when and what we ate the previous day that the food gaps show up. Those who are overweight can be assured that the diet will help them lose weight and decrease their bloatedness. But those who are below ideal weight and very weight conscious may be best advised to keep off the scales entirely and rely only on the doctor's scales.

I always weigh and measure my patients, and then refer to the Society of Actuaries tables, which give the ideal health weight consistent with age and height. Too many women do not appreciate that the ideal weight increases with age. Menopausal women like to remain at their teenage weight, but alas! Nature has decided otherwise.

If a vaginal discharge, itching, or a history of recurrent thrush is reported, then it is wise to have a vaginal swab tested to ensure that thrush does not develop or become exacerbated when progesterone is used. Today, treatment of thrush is simple enough: with just one capsule of Diflucan 150 mg for the patient and her partner, all is well in a few days.

SLEEP PATTERN

The usual type and duration of sleep also need discussion. The average woman needs eight hours of bed rest, but many women with PMS need more. In a busy life, it is all too easy to try to manage on seven hours during the week and then enjoy the luxury of sleeping in on the weekend. Often a short discussion of the need for adequate sleep each night helps solve many problems. We all need horizontal bed rest at night, because this is when the kidneys work extra well. It does not really matter whether we are conscious or sleeping soundly: the kidneys still work extra well while we are horizontal. So if you wake up at night, don't go walking about the house or making a cup of tea. Worse still, never take a sleeping tablet in the middle of the night. Remember that children and adults all wake up at night, but they usually turn over and then forget that they have ever woken up. It is only as we get older that we tend to notice the waking, start worrying, and fear that we will be tired and depressed the next day. Instead, if you wake, continue to lie peacefully, and, ideally, think happy thoughts, plan your dream holiday or wardrobe, or decide how you will spend your lottery millions. You may be happiest listening to the radio or comforting music. Train your mind to switch off from problems during the night, and give yourself a set half-hour each day for problem solving and thinking about your worries.

LIFESTYLE

With women now working both outside and in the home, too many imagine that they no longer deserve any rest during the day. Working men always break at midday, have some food, relax, and socialize, and when they return home after a day's hard work they relax. Women, on the other hand, tend to use the lunch break to catch up on the shopping, and as soon as they get home busy themselves with preparing, eating, and clearing up for the next meal. Some even start ironing, cleaning, or other necessary housework. They seem to regard a short break or relaxation during the day as a sign of laziness. It is only when the day's pattern is examined closely that many realize that if they managed differently, they too could put their feet up and rest for the odd half-hour before starting work again. An eight-hour workday would be a luxury to many women.

SMOKING

It has been shown in rats that smoking lowers the blood progesterone level. Those who have been working for years with sufferers of PMS will agree that women's PMS symptoms are relieved when they stop smoking. It is always worth discussing smoking, because it may be just the right time and a new reason to stop the habit.

TREATMENT OF MENSTRUAL MAGNIFICATION

When there is a vast increase in the severity of symptoms from the follicular phase to the premenstruum, this constitutes the diagnosis of *menstrual magnification* or *menstrual distress*. Symptoms in the follicular phase can vary from 5 percent to 95 percent, and often the simple lifestyle changes already mentioned may reduce the follicular phase symptoms, transferring the diagnosis to PMS. Generally speaking, if the menstrual chart shows the severity of follicular symptoms is less than 50 percent, then it is worth giving the full treatment for PMS. However, the woman must appreciate that she does not have a diagnosis of PMS, and as shown in Figure 49 (page 224), she is not so likely to benefit from the Three-Hourly Starch Diet. Also, it is important that she not volunteer for clinical trials on PMS. If 50 percent of symptoms are present throughout the cycle, then further investigations into the cause of her problems are indicated.

TREATMENT OF SINGLE SYMPTOMS

If there appears to be only one severe symptom, then it is best to first try conventional treatment for that symptom. It is in this category that psychiatrists treat premenstrual tension, which is discussed in chapter 26.

Other examples of a single symptom responding to well-recognized treatment for that symptom include using a nasal spray to ease premenstrual rhinitis, or an inhaler for premenstrual asthma. Some types of facial acne and rosacea respond well to a course of oxytetracycline.

TREATMENTS NEVER EVALUATED

In the early 1980s, the Boston PMS clinic was successfully using British progesterone suppositories (Cyclogest) when the FDA reminded them that the drug had not been licensed in America, so must not be imported. This brought a rush of unorthodox medications, which have never been evaluated. While they may benefit the general health of both men and women, there is no evidence that they are valuable in the treatment of PMS. Nor is there any evidence of a deficiency of the preparation during the premenstruum The list includes garlic tablets, St. John's Wort, magnesium, Chinese herbs, and various vitamin and mineral preparations.

VITAMIN B-6

Vitamin B-6, or pyridoxine, has frequently been advised for PMS, among other conditions. In 1983, Schaumberg and his colleagues in New York reported in the *New England Journal of Medicine* seven cases of people, some wheelchair-bound, with severe nerve damage due to excessive doses of vitamin B-6. Schaumberg, a neurologist, had previously studied the nerves of dogs and rats when trying to find a cure for peripheral neuritis, which is a chronic and painful condition prevalent in diabetics and alcoholics. Schaumberg showed, using microscopic studies, that an overdose of vitamin B-6 caused the

same type of degeneration of nerve endings in humans, causing them to suffer peripheral neuritis.

In 1987, the paper "Characteristics of Pyridoxine
Overdose Neuropathy Syndrome" in *Acta Neurologica
Scandinavia*, which I co-authored with my son, Dr. Michael
Dalton, described 172 women all currently taking at least 50
mg daily of vitamin B-6 and with a raised pyridoxine blood
level. It won the Cullen Nutrition Prize at the Royal Free
Hospital Medical School, University of London. The paper
showed that among these 172 women with high pyridoxine
blood levels, 60 percent already had signs of nerve damage.
The damage occurred after taking the vitamin for six months
or more, continuously or intermittently. The duration was
more important than the actual dose. The symptoms of overdose included pins and needles in the arms and legs, supersen-
sitivity or burning of the skin, muscle weakness, shooting
pains, and generalized itching (see Figure 48).

In 1990, Doctors Kleinjen, Ter Rier, and Knipschild in the
Netherlands did a metanalysis of all the published controlled trials in which vitamin B-6 had been used as treatment for PMS,
and they could find no evidence of beneficial effect. However,
the sale of vitamin B-6 continued to be advocated for PMS. In
Europe, apart from Britain and the Netherlands, doses of vitamin
B-6 over 10 mg must be medically prescribed. Vitamin B-6 is not
a drug licensed by the FDA, but rather a food controlled by the
Department of Agriculture. In May 1997, when the Labor government was elected in Britain, one of their first proposals was to
limit over-the-counter sales of vitamin B-6 to 10 mg tablets.
Such a regulation would have meant a disastrous loss of revenue
for health food stores, estimated at £34 million, so they formed a
powerful lobby group to fight back. Our article of 1987 was the
only medical publication to have reported raised pyridoxine
blood levels in women, so the findings came under scrutiny. To
substantiate our original findings, we wrote to all the 172 women
asking how their health had been in the last ten years and if they
had any new medical diagnosis. They were compared with an

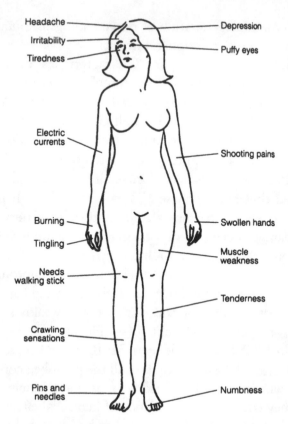

Figure 48   Symptoms of vitamin B-6 overdose

equal number of women who had had any blood test in the same practice in 1986 or 1987 and who had *not* taken vitamin B-6. The results were a shock to us and to the government. Compared with the vitamin B-6 takers, those who had never taken vitamin B-6 had had better health and fewer deaths in the previous ten years. Moreover, one-third of the vitamin B-6 takers had developed an autoimmune disease, such as thyroid disease, diabetes, lupus, rheumatoid arthritis, or Sjögrens syndrome. This finding caused the government to stop any further legislation while appointing an expert committee to look into the problem and report within two years. The government reminded the public that it still recommended 10 mg daily as the limit.

23

··*

Counseling for PMS

Wendy Holton

It is important to remember that premenstrual syndrome is a whole collection of very different symptoms, some physical and others psychological. PMS Help, a national charity in Britain, surveyed their members' reporting of symptoms. They found that the average number of premenstrual symptoms reported was seven, though some women reported as many as thirteen different symptoms recurring each month before menstruation. The seven symptoms usually reported included both physical and psychological symptoms, but no two members surveyed had the same seven. The variations were endless.

With seven symptoms, trying to treat each symptom individually is not recommended. Can you imagine treating the bloatedness with water pills, the headache with analgesics, the weight gain by calorie reduction, the dermatitis with steroidal creams, the sore throat with lozenges, the tension with aggression therapy, and the indecisiveness with assertiveness training? Any woman in this scenario would find herself spinning with such a collection of different treatments.

As discussed earlier, it is the timing and not the symptoms that clinches the diagnosis of PMS, and its treatment needs to cover the whole spectrum of symptoms, not each symptom individually. Therefore, although psychological help may, in some cases, aid the psychological symptoms, it is unlikely to bring relief for the physical symptoms which are almost certainly present too.

The recommended first step in relief of PMS symptoms is dietary. I recommend following the Three-Hourly Starch Diet, which ensures that you have some starchy food every three hours of your waking day, always within an hour of waking and an hour before going to bed at night. Starchy foods are any that contain wheat, rice, oats, potato, corn, or rye. These need to be combined with a good general diet for good health. You will find your symptoms will start to ease within days of sticking rigidly to this diet. Full details are contained in chapter 24.

So is there a place for counseling within the treatment of PMS? On its own, counseling will not relieve PMS; however, there is a place for it in some cases, either simultaneously with the diet and, if necessary, hormonal medication, or after the PMS has been controlled. Whatever type of counseling you consider, it should always be with a trained, reputable counselor.

Whatever the problem in today's society, there always seems to be a call for counseling, almost with the assumption that a counselor can make the problem vanish. Unfortunately, counseling cannot make anything vanish, but it can help the sufferer to talk about the problem, and in that talking perhaps find a way in which the situation can be managed less painfully.

There are many different types of counseling strategies. Some of these prove more useful than others in helping sufferers of premenstrual syndrome who wish to combine therapy with their treatment program.

Take, for example, those who in the days prior to menstruation experience a buildup of anger, which they try to control as best they can, to avoid the volcanic explosion that so regularly occurs. In this situation, methods that facilitate expressing the anger and talking from the other's place may prove helpful. However, this should be done only under the supervision of a trained counselor.

Once PMS symptoms are relieved by other means and life improves, there also may be a place for counseling. It can help a woman to deal with her guilt about the damage she may have done to relationships, and harmful actions and words, particularly those directed at family and close friends. Words said in anger or sarcasm do not just disappear as PMS symptoms do, when menstruation occurs and the speaker is feeling normal again. The hurt caused can sometimes fester until a friendship or relationship is destroyed. In these cases, counseling to cope with the aftereffects of the PMS is a natural step, along with treatment to ensure that the eruption does not recur the next month or the month after that.

Just as the variety of symptoms is endless, the effects of those symptoms can also be wide-ranging, but it is the psychological symptoms, combined with violent acts, which afterward bring remorse and guilt. In these circumstances, counseling is advantageous in helping to come to terms with the guilt and conflict of emotions thus caused.

The realization that it was your untreated PMS that was at the root of a physical assault on a child, partner, or animal can take a long time to accept and come to terms with. The realization that it was your PMS that led to an injury in a car and subsequent financial loss may leave unresolved or repressed guilt. The desire to be slim may lead to an unrealistic diet with long food gaps, which in turn can cause the anguish of many months or even years of premenstrual syndrome. Once normalcy has returned, the healthy woman may be able to see her PMS as self-inflicted and to realize that her own selfishness, although unacknowledged at the time, was a possible cause. These are all areas in which counseling can be beneficial—but only once the initial premenstrual syndrome has been controlled with diet and, if necessary, medication. If PMS continues untreated and recurs regularly, counseling alone is only a kind of Band-Aid to stop the initial bleeding; it will not bring long-term relief.

Programs like the NLP (Neuro-Linguistic Programming) techniques pioneered by Richard Bandler and John Grinder can often be of assistance in increasing a woman's confidence. They can empower her if she lacks confidence and help her to sail through her low self-esteem days. By using basic stress relief techniques for behavior change, she is able to bring up positive thoughts at those times when negativity takes over.

STRESS RELIEF

Basic stress-relief techniques need to be taught to women suffering from PMS, because stress so often exacerbates premenstrual symptoms, causing far greater problems than are necessary. The following stress busters are simple but extremely effective—even non-PMS sufferers can benefit from them.

Breathing

Sit quietly and comfortably in a straight-back chair, such as a dining room chair, and breathe deeply and gently. Be sure that you exhale all the air in your lungs before breathing in deeply and then exhaling again. You will feel your diaphragm moving up and down and a calmness will gently envelop you. As you continue breathing deeply, you will notice a sensation of relaxation flow through you. You need only devote a couple of minutes a day to training yourself to breathe deeply and gently.

Progressive Muscle Relaxation

Lie on the floor or on a firm bed, or sit in a straight-back chair. Take a few deep and gentle breaths until you are in a calm state. Clench your toes and count to five, then relax. Repeat this five times. Next, contract the muscles in your feet and ankles and hold them tight for a count of five before relaxing them. When you have repeated this five times, move to your calf muscles, hold them tight for a count of five before relaxing, and repeat this five times. And so on through the knees, thighs, and buttocks, before you move to the fingers, wrists, forearms, upper arms, shoulders, and so on, each time tensing that group of muscles for a count of five before relaxing them, repeating each exercise five times. You then can move to the face, screwing up the eyes, tensing the lips and cheeks, and frowning. When you have tensed and relaxed all the groups of muscles you can think of, lie or sit still and breathe gently, in a fully relaxed state, for at least five minutes before gently feeling each set of muscles as you get up. Don't rush. Enjoy the feeling of relaxation and lightness.

Visualizing

If a particular problem is causing you unnecessary concern and stress, it may get out of proportion and dominate your life. Here is an exercise you can try in these cases. Sit in a comfortable position, gently close your eyes, and picture the problem. Take some time to survey it as a picture. Mentally place a frame around the picture so that it looks like a postcard then move the postcard into the background until it diminishes in size. Clear the postcard from your mind and visualize a relaxing scene, perhaps a landscape, a sunny beach, or a gentle stream flowing through a green meadow. Put a frame around this, your "master picture," to make a postcard. Move this postcard around so that the initial problem postcard is visible at the same time before bringing the master postcard back into focus and letting the problem one shrink in proportion or disappear.

Sleep

Restful sleep is very important, yet so often people find themselves tossing and turning, unable to sleep. If this is your problem, the first step is to make sure that you have eaten some starchy food within the past hour. If you have and are still unable fall asleep, a good way to induce the relaxed state and subsequent sleep is to lie comfortably in your usual sleep position. With your eyes closed, picture a blackboard. In your

mind's eye, draw the number 99 on it, and place a border
around the number. Look at the number for a second or two
and then wipe the number and border away. Then draw the
number 98 with a border, look at it, then wipe it away too. Do
the same with the number 97, and so on in descending order,
till you drop off to sleep. You will be surprised how the mind
will become bored and relaxed, and sleep will overcome you.

Exercise

For general good health, it is essential to exercise. We all need
some physical activity, be it walking, dancing, jogging, aero-
bics, swimming, a game of racquetball, or climbing a rock face.
The range of opportunities is endless, and many are free or
quite inexpensive. Choose the type of exercise you enjoy and
participate in it at least three times a week for approximately
twenty minutes each time.

Although you may think you don't have time, it will surprise you how quickly you will gain time by exercising. If you
really do not have an opportunity to start exercising, how
about giving up the elevator and walking up and down the
stairs? Or park your car at the far end of the parking lot and
walk to the shops or to your office—when it is safe to do so, of
course. All these simple exercises help to relieve stress and will
benefit the majority of PMS sufferers.

24

_____ ?❧ _____

The Three-Hourly Starch Diet

It is the molecular biologists who demonstrated the unique characteristics of progesterone receptors and showed that a progesterone receptor cannot transport, or bind to, a molecule of progesterone if there has been a drop in blood sugar (Figure 49).

A drop in blood sugar causes a release of adrenaline, which
automatically moves sugar from cells into the blood, raising the
blood sugar level. This is one of Nature's clever tricks to ensure
that our blood sugar remains within optimum limits at all times.
All cells contain sugar, and if sugar goes into the blood, water
replaces it and enters the cell. The cells swell up, causing a feeling of bloatedness, and later, weight gain. Furthermore, adrenaline is the hormone of "fight, flight, and fright" and therefore con-
tributes to the tension that PMS patients experience (Figure 50).

One recent finding has been that the blood level
of progesterone drops after a large meal (Figure 51), a discovery which again emphasizes the need for women with PMS to
eat smaller amounts at any one time, but to eat more often.

This means that for PMS sufferers, the first essential is to
ensure there is no drop in the blood sugar level, which occurs
when there has been a long interval between meals. Men can
easily go up to eight hours without food; they are "gorgers." But
for healthy women the interval is shorter, averaging five hours,
because they are "grazers." Unfortunately, those suffering from

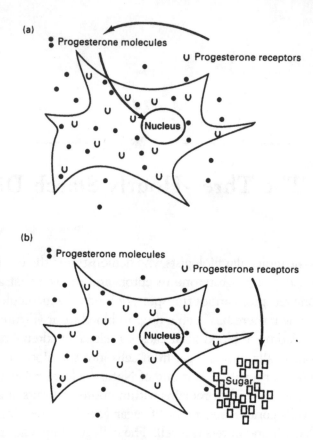

Figure 49   Action of progesterone receptors

PMS need to eat every three hours. This is the reason for the Three-Hourly Starch Diet, which by itself will relieve many of the symptoms of PMS; without this diet, progesterone is not effective.

RULES OF THE THREE-HOURLY STARCH DIET

Divide the day's starchy food so that you eat small starchy snacks every three hours during the waking hours and within one hour of waking and retiring to bed. Meanwhile, continue with a healthy diet with adequate protein and plenty of fruit and vegetables. Starchy foods are those containing wheat,

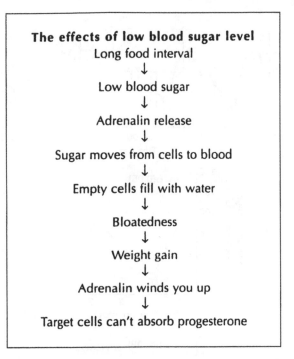

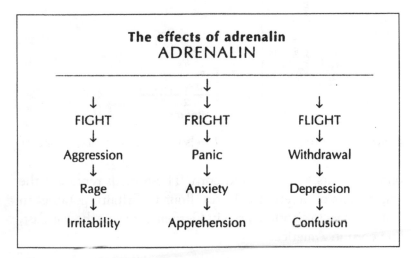

Figure 50   The effects of low blood sugar and adrenaline

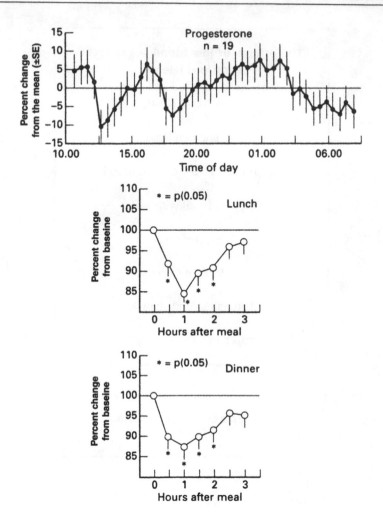

Figure 51   Progesterone blood levels in relation to food intake

potatoes, oats, rice, rye, and corn. These foods represent the staple diets of different cultures: flour in Britain, potatoes in Ireland, oats in Scotland, rye in Germany, rice in the Far East, and corn in America.

The Three-Hourly Starch Diet

- Eat small starchy snacks every three hours during the waking hours.

- Always eat a starchy snack within an hour of rising.
- Always eat a starchy snack within an hour of going to bed.
- Continue on the diet throughout the menstrual cycle.
- Continue eating a healthy, varied, and nutritious diet.

It takes at least seven days before the benefit of frequent eating is appreciated, and unfortunately, if there are long gaps between eating or snacking it will take up to seven days to recover. One excited responder to the diet wrote,

> The answer to all my suffering and irritability lies in my kitchen.

It may be difficult initially, but the diet soon becomes a habit, and then it is no longer necessary to keep your eye on your watch. It is important to have an emergency snack handy in your handbag, in your car, and hidden in the office. It is no good giving the excuse that you are not allowed to eat at work: under the law you are allowed to take a ten-minute break at least every four hours, so don't let your supervisor bully you. If you are going into a meeting or conference that might clash with your nibble time, then always eat just before you go into the conference room. It does not matter if you eat every hour or two, as long as you don't wait longer than three hours. When you go out to a sumptuous meal, it is still possible to continue with the diet, by choosing an appetizer and dessert that contains no starch and eating just a small portion of potatoes, rice, or pasta, while enjoying the meat, fish, and vegetables of the main dish.

EATING HABITS FIFTY YEARS AGO

In 1948, the first six women who responded to progesterone for PMS were all housewives looking after children. They spent much of their time in the kitchen cooking cakes, pastries, stews, and casseroles. Good cooks always taste, so they would have been nibbling all day. The well-heeled ladies had their breakfast, morning coffee, lunch, afternoon tea, supper, and a snack before bed to prevent "night starvation." There were large family meals, with the matriarch serving from the head of the table, giving hearty helpings to the men and smaller portions to the women. A woman's place was in the home. This was before almost all women went to work regardless of whether they had children or not. It was before the Twiggy era, and before health education advised everyone to lose weight. Three meals a day was the norm. There were no fast foods, no convenience food, no microwaves, and no eating before the TV. Today, the food portions are usually of equal size for both men and women. This probably explains the success with progesterone in the early years, when more women were eating every three hours, or at least more frequently than now.

EFFECTIVENESS OF THE THREE-HOURLY STARCH DIET

In 1992 I published a paper with Wendy Holton in *Stress Medicine*. It discussed the diets of eighty-four women with

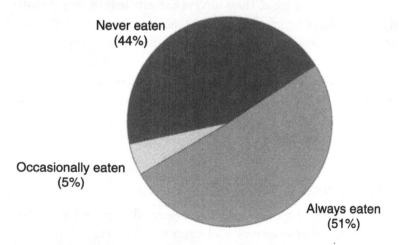

Figure 52   PMS sufferers who eat breakfast

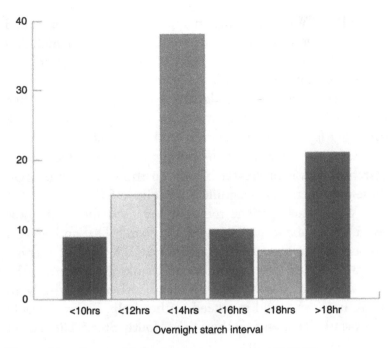

Figure 53 Overnight food gaps in women with PMS

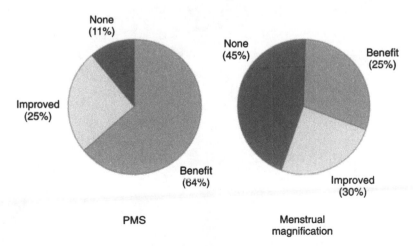

Figure 54 Effect of Three-Hourly Starch Diet on PMS and menstrual magnification

severe PMS. While awaiting an appointment, the women had been sent seven diet forms and asked to complete them during each of the next seven days. The results showed that only 51 percent regularly ate breakfast (Figure 52).

There were also long daytime food gaps, averaging five hours or more, and long overnight food gaps. Ideally, the overnight fast should not exceed ten hours (Figure 53).

Of equal interest was the finding that the Three-Hourly Starch Diet was of greater benefit to those with PMS than those with menstrual magnification (Figure 54).

When each patient returned her food forms, she was given advice about the Three-Hourly Starch Diet and advised to continue with it until her appointment. During the interval, several canceled their appointment, thanking us, because the diet alone had solved their problems; others came only to thank us, as they did not need further help. Today, I would firmly start all patients on the Three-Hourly Starch Diet before prescribing progesterone.

25

Rules of Progesterone Treatment

There is a vast gulf between scientists, who are forever discovering new facts about progesterone and progesterone receptors, and clinicians, most of whom have not updated their knowledge and appreciate neither the difference between progesterone and progestogens, nor the fact that progestogens lower progesterone blood levels. Many psychiatrists have never studied hormone therapy, even in their medical training, so perhaps they may be excused for only being able to see PMS as a psychiatric problem rather than as a problem of unbalanced hormonal receptors.

Progesterone therapy should be accompanied by regular menstrual and symptomatic recording, so that the benefit, or otherwise, of treatment is obvious. Ideally the patient should already have been on the Three-Hourly Starch Diet for a minimum of seven days, and questions about the diet eaten the previous day should be noted and discussed, with any slight errors corrected.

Before starting progesterone treatment:

- Ensure that the patient is using, and continues to use, a menstrual chart competently (see pages 17–19).

- Ensure that the patient understands the relationship of smoking, alcohol consumption, and sleep deficit to PMS.
- Ensure that the patient is not on the Pill, HRT, or medication containing progestogen or vitamin B-6.
- Ensure that the patient has maintained the Three-Hourly Starch Diet for at least one week and understands the reasons for continuing with it.
- Ensure that no thrush infection is present.

INDIVIDUAL VARIATION OF PROGESTERONE ABSORPTION

Dr. Maureen Dalton and her team at St. James's University Hospital, Leeds, studied the effect of a single dose of 50 mg progesterone in the follicular phase on nineteen healthy women who received either intramuscular, vaginal, oral, or nasal administration. A marked individual variation was evident in the peak concentration, the peak time, and the level after two hours. Intramuscular progesterone had the best absorption, and it was only when progesterone was used intramuscularly that there was any correlation between body weight and progesterone levels—it was most effective in those of thin build.

The effectiveness of progesterone depends on the route of administration and the precise cells intended to receive progesterone. In PMS it is the systemic cells, for instance, those of the brain, bones, and lungs, that need progesterone. The most effective route for PMS is by intramuscular injections of progesterone 50 or 100 mg into the buttocks, either daily or on alternate days. Nasal absorption is the least effective.

Rectal suppositories of progesterone 400 mg dissolved in inert wax are effective in raising the progesterone blood level for between four and eighteen hours, which means they must be used at least twice daily, although as individuals are all different, some may need up to six daily. The minimum dose for PMS is twice daily with suppositories of 400 mg.

Vaginal progesterone suppositories may be used in the same dose levels for PMS. The wax will melt at body temperature and is rather messy, but this can be eased by the use of sanitary protection or a panty liner at the time of insertion, followed twenty to thirty minutes later by a wipe or wash, when all the progesterone will have been absorbed. Dr. D. De Ziegler and his colleagues at the Columbia Laboratories in Paris have recently shown that there is a first-pass route for progesterone from the vagina to the endometrium, which is several times higher than the route from the vagina to systemic circulation. Thus, lower doses of progesterone vaginal suppositories can be used when the progesterone is needed directly on the endometrial lining of the womb for in vitro fertilization, early pregnancy, and certain gynecological conditions.

If progesterone is administered orally, it passes from the gut via the portal blood system to the liver, where it is metabolized before reaching the systemic blood circulation. So oral administration is not very helpful for PMS.

There is currently uncertainty about systemic absorption through the skin. There has been a failure in England to demonstrate any absorption, even of micronized progesterone. A sample of progesterone cream sent for testing in London in 1998 was found to contain no progesterone and was described as an "error." In view of the apparently good results obtained in California, a possible answer may be the state's tropical climate in which the skin pores are continually open. Or perhaps a new preparation is in use containing better absorptive properties. Progesterone cream is helpful if applied locally, especially for wrinkles. It is not licensed for use in England.

INDICATIONS FOR PROGESTERONE INJECTIONS

Intramuscular progesterone is the most effective treatment for PMS, so it should be the first choice for those at risk of severe premenstrual symptoms, such as asthma, suicide, assault, or alcoholic bouts, or those at risk of a prison sentence following recurrent conflicts with the law. If treatment with suppositories has failed or brought insufficient relief, injections should be used for those with recurrent symptoms interfering with their normal working capacity and lifestyle, as well as for those with problems arising from marital or domestic stress, especially if children are involved. If daily supervision is required, as with those at risk of suicide, child abuse, or alcoholic bouts, then injections given by a responsible individual are preferred. Nurses in hospitals and prisons usually prefer to use injections rather than suppositories, the use of which is not so easily supervised.

The injections should be given into the buttocks, where there are clumps of fat cells between the muscle fibers, which go in all directions. The progesterone in oil first passes to the fat cells and is then slowly transferred to the blood. The injections may be given anywhere in the buttocks where there is a one-inch pinch of fat, but never in the thighs or deltoid muscle. In nonpregnant women, the dose rarely needs to exceed 100 mg daily, but suppositories, used rectally or vaginally, may supplement the dose.

The injection should never be given in an area that is hot, hard, or painful, a sign that a previous injection has not yet been fully absorbed into the blood. If the injections is given by a nurse, a partner, or a friend, it is best if the patient stands upright, feet a foot apart, with toes turned inward. If the patient injects herself, she may sit down and inject into her upper buttocks, and at other times lean against a table and slide the syringe along the surface so that it goes in at right angles. By bending her knees at varying angles, she can ensure that she does not inject into the same spot twice. The best time for an injection is immediately before a nice, long laze in the bath, which gives an opportunity for the progesterone to move from the fat cells into the blood.

PROGESTERONE SUPPOSITORIES

The minimum dose of progesterone suppositories is 400 mg twice daily, but the dose may be increased up to 400 mg six times daily, although there must always be a minimum of two hours between insertions. Women usually try both vaginal and rectal insertions and then determine their preference. Injections and suppositories can be alternated, using injections and suppositories on alternate days, or suppositories in the morning and injections in the evening.

Those who have had many children, those of slim build, and those who have previously suffered from preeclampsia or postnatal depression usually require higher doses. Adjustment of medication is usually necessary after a pregnancy, and if all has been normal, progesterone may no longer be required.

Once there has been relief of all premenstrual symptoms for three months, the dose may be gradually reduced, either by starting a day or two later each month or by reducing the dose each month, while continuing to start the course on Day 14.

Women over forty are likely to require progesterone until the menopause, while those under twenty-five may need progesterone for only six to nine months.

Occasionally, for some women, progesterone may cause lengthening of the usual cycle, in which case, stopping progesterone two days before the time of normal menstruation is usually effective. Other women may find that progesterone therapy shortens their normal cycle; they can be helped by starting future courses of progesterone a couple of days later. If progesterone has been started in the follicular phase, there may be slight spotting at ovulation. This is of no significance if other causes of erratic bleeding have been eliminated. If a dose or two of progesterone has been forgotten, menstruation may start unexpectedly. Erratic users tend to have erratic cycles.

USER-FRIENDLY PROGESTERONE

There are no drug interactions with progesterone, which is a natural hormone produced in massive amounts during pregnancy. Patients already on drug therapy, such as antidepressants, tranquilizers, beta-blockers, or anticonvulsants, may continue on their normal dose when starting progesterone and then gradually reduce their other medication. Any other medication should always be gradually reduced after menstruation. Progesterone may occasionally be given with progestogens, as for example in cases of endometriosis. A general urticarial rash following a progesterone injection is very rare, and is caused by the oil in which the progesterone is dissolved, so treatment can be continued with suppositories.

Professor Jerilyn Prior has shown that progesterone is as effective as estrogen in the treatment of osteoporosis. Progesterone may be used to assist conception and contraception.

Other Indications for Progesterone Therapy

- In vitro fertilization
- Habitual abortion, if cause is not chromosomal or anatomical
- Morning sickness and symptoms of early pregnancy
- Symptoms of mid-pregnancy and the prevention of preeclampsia
- Prevention of postnatal depression
- Contraception in those unable to tolerate hormonal contraception
- Menopause: Progesterone may be used instead of progestogens to promote cyclical bleeding while on estrogen replacement therapy
- Prevention of osteoporosis

26

---- ❧ ----

Psychiatric Treatment

Psychiatric PMS symptoms are caused by abnormalities of brain chemistry, and we now know that they can be helped by chemicals aimed at correcting the abnormalities. Psychiatric treatment is best for those PMS sufferers whose only symptoms are premenstrual tension or other psychiatric symptoms, but who have no physical symptoms. It may be preferred by those who do not want to follow the Three-Hourly Starch Diet required for progesterone treatment, as well as by those with menstrual magnification, who have psychiatric symptoms throughout the month but are free from physical symptoms.

PREMENSTRUAL TENSION

The three predominant symptoms in premenstrual tension are depression, irritability, and lethargy. Unfortunately, tricyclic antidepressants will relieve the depression but increase the lethargy. Tranquilizers will relieve the irritability but increase the lethargy. Amphetamines will relieve the lethargy but increase the irritability. Therefore, premenstrual tension will not be eased by any single class of the most popular psychiatric medications.

237

SELECTIVE SEROTONIN REUPTAKE INHIBITORS

Prozac was the forerunner of a new group of psychiatric drugs known as the selective serotonin reuptake inhibitors (SSRIs). Although there were initial problems with Prozac, these have been ironed out over the last five years, and many new and better SSRIs have been developed. These have fewer side effects but remain equally effective, and include fluoxitine, paroxitine, and sertraline. Rather than being antidepressants, they act more like antianxiety drugs. As early as 1984 Doctors Taylor, Matthew, and Beng noted that serotonin, a neurotransmitter in the brain, was at a low level in the platelets of premenstrual tension sufferers. PMS women with tension symptoms but no physical symptoms certainly benefit from SSRIs. Patients are best started initially on half a dose daily for one week, during which they personally discover the best time of day to take the medication. Some may find the tablet causes insomnia and therefore is best taken on waking. Others may find that taking the tablet on rising causes nausea and drowsiness that last all day, and they are advised to take the tablet at night. We are all different in our optimum timing for SSRIs. Once the patient has determined the best time to take the tablet, the dose can be doubled. She should continue on that dose for at least two weeks before attempting to increase the dose, which will probably not be necessary. If it is effective for one cycle, then future doses need be given only from ovulation until menstruation, being limited to the time of the premenstrual symptoms. Once my patients have started, I prefer that they continue the medication for a full six months, and then make a trial reduction to half a dose. Often the nuclei of the brain cells have learned by then to perform their correct

---

PROGESTERONE
is a
NATURAL MONOAMINE OXIDASE INHIBITOR

biochemical task, and after another month the SSRIs can be stopped without a recurrence of PMS symptoms.

MONOAMINE OXIDASE INHIBITORS

Monoamine oxidase inhibitors (MAOIs) are another group of powerful antidepressants that do not take long to work that work faster than and are especially useful in atypical (nontypical) depression. Two American doctors, Shader and Goldblatt, suggested the acronym TROUBLE to describe patients most likely to benefit from MAOIs. It stands for:

T = Trouble
R = Regressive (going downhill)
O = Overanxious
U = Unstable
B = Bulimic
L = Labile (mood swings)
E = Episodic (good and bad times)

Although effective, MAOIs have severe reactions with certain foods, so patients must be warned never to eat cheese or meat extracts or drink red wine, and to avoid certain medications. It can be fatal for the patient to disobey the dietary restrictions. Fortunately, since the introduction of SSRIs, the use of MAOIs has diminished.

In 1991, Dr. Zuspan and his team of molecular biologists at the University of Chicago showed, by using a culture of placental cells, that progesterone has an inhibitory effect on monoamine oxidase; in short, they demonstrated that progesterone is a natural monoamine oxidase inhibitor (MAOI), and like MAOIs, it inhibits the accumulation of monoamine oxidase in the brain.

PREMENSTRUAL PSYCHOSIS

Premenstrual psychosis is usually short-lived, lasting only a day or two. However, the presence of hallucinations, delusions, disorientation, and confusion usually cause it to be brought to the attention of a psychiatrist early in an episode, which may lead to compulsory detention of the patient in a hospital. Psychiatrists have effective antipsychotic drugs, which quickly normalize a patient. Once menstruation starts, within a day or two the patient may be discharged. If another episode of psychosis occurs the following month, the patient will be kept in the hospital longer and may be discharged on antipsychotic medication, such as is used for schizophrenia. After three or more episodes, if the psychotic episodes are not recognized as being related to menstruation, long-term medication is the usual outcome. Long-term antipsychotic medication brings with it general mental dullness and the risk of tardive dyskinesia or parkinsonism.

In 1998, I was asked to see Emma, a seventeen-year-old, in custody for arson. Her mother had alerted the lawyers to the possibility of PMS and provided details of four previous overdose attempts, which had all occurred premenstrually. Emma had been admitted to the secure unit of a mental hospital for four months, but four days before my visit she had been transferred back to prison, as she was not considered to have a psychiatric illness. She had been given antipsychotic medication in the hospital; the precise type or dosage was unknown to me, but she had the very worst case of parkinsonism I had ever seen. My report to the court read:

> She was brought in assisted by two nurses. She was shuffling, her feet never leaving the ground. The nurses helped her into the chair in front of my desk. She sat bent over, with her forearms on the desk and her head leaning on her hands, which were holding wet tissues. She had a continuous shake of the whole body, with a never-ending drip of saliva from her mouth to her hands, tissues, or desk. This shaking and salivation continued throughout the interview. Eye contact was impossible, although there were a few momentary occasions when she lifted her head slightly and her eyes became visible, and her rigid face could be seen. Her left forearm was bandaged, because she had scalded her arm under boiling water some three days earlier.

27

———————— ❧ ————————

Pregnancy and Postnatal Depression

Considering the important role the pregnancy hormone progesterone plays in PMS, it is not surprising that pregnancy also plays an important role for those suffering from PMS. Problems related to PMS may arise before, during, or after a pregnancy. Indeed, four out of five women who suffer from either preeclampsia or postnatal depression are likely to be left with moderate to severe PMS. Contraception is a source of concern to women who suffer from PMS, because hormonal contraceptives (either pills, injections, or implants) and bilateral tubal surgery increase PMS.

For our great-grandparents it was a matter of luck how many children arrived, and when. Those days have long since passed, and today it is a question of "Shall we?" "When?" or "Why haven't we?" Our medical resources seem to be shared equally between helping people to conceive and helping people to avoid pregnancy.

CONCEPTION

The release of an egg at ovulation is the first essential to conception, and it is only during the next twenty-four hours or so that conception is possible. This may cause difficulty in women who travel much, or whose partner is frequently away from home, for they need to calculate their fertile days with care. Women who suffer from or have had spasmodic dysmenorrhea already know that for them ovulation occurs regularly. Women suffering from PMS can usually conceive easily, because they are aware of their fertile times. However, if symptoms such as migraines or rage become acute at ovulation, then they may avoid intercourse at the very time that successful conception is likely.

Women for whom pregnancy is possible, as well as those positively anxious to conceive, are advised to keep a regular temperature and menstrual chart (see page 18). Those hoping for success may also want to keep a daily temperature chart, which in many cases will show the precise day of ovulation, but such charts are not infallible and are difficult to interpret. The woman should take her temperature daily for at least two minutes before she gets out of bed in the morning and record the reading on a temperature chart. The temperature and menstrual charts should also note the days of intercourse, for although this may occur at least twenty times during a month, if it does not include the day of ovulation, pregnancy may be impossible. If pregnancy has occurred, the temperature remains raised after the day of the expected menstruation. (Full details for temperature charting are covered in *The Fertility Awareness Handbook* by Barbara Kass-Annese and Hal Danzer, M.D; Alameda, CA: Hunter House, 1992, 6th ed.)

Women receiving progesterone for PMS should start their course after ovulation. They may recognize ovulation by the slight abdominal pain in one side of the lower abdomen, by the change in vaginal discharge, or by the change in their morning temperature. In these cases timing their progesterone is easy. Otherwise, they should start ten or twelve days before the expected day of the next menstruation. There are also ovulation kits on the market that are simple to use and will accurately pinpoint the day of ovulation. Progesterone should be continued once pregnancy has been confirmed and continued if there are any unpleasant pregnancy symptoms, such as nausea, tiredness, headache, or depression. If necessary, the dose of progesterone can be increased until all pregnancy symptoms subside.

If you have any doubts as to whether ovulation is actually occurring and you are anxious to become pregnant, then it is wise to seek medical advice. There are drugs to stimulate ovulation. Failure to ovulate is not the only cause of failure to conceive, so if pregnancy does not come when planned, a visit to a gynecologist is advised.

Progesterone is used in *in vitro fertilization*, when the embryo is replaced for the early months of pregnancy, and also if there is a history of defective luteal phase or habitual abortion. Progesterone is also helpful for those suffering from morning sickness or vomiting in early pregnancy. This is because the placenta is not yet fully formed and is not producing sufficient progesterone. The symptoms usually pass by the sixteenth to twentieth week of pregnancy.

PLACENTAL PROGESTERONE

Immediately after conception, hormonal changes occur and a new organ, the placenta, is formed in the womb. The placenta is the center of hormonal activity between the mother and her developing baby. It passes nutrients to, supplies oxygen to, and removes waste from the baby. The placenta produces massive amounts of progesterone, and it is usually fully formed by the fourth month. In the early days of pregnancy, a woman may experience nausea and vomiting, often called "morning sickness"; the medical term for this is *hyperemesis*. This is a sign that the ovarian progesterone is insufficient and the placenta is not yet secreting enough progesterone, so progesterone may be given to ease the symptoms. The rules of progesterone treatment are still important, and strict adherence to the Three-Hourly Starch Diet may be sufficient to relieve these symptoms of the early stages of pregnancy (see page 223).

Once the placenta is fully formed, it produces some forty times the normal progesterone level found at the peak of the luteal phase of a menstrual cycle. This is the time that most women with PMS suddenly blossom, feeling better than they have ever felt. Indeed, some ten to twenty years later they may fondly recall those healthy days during their pregnancy when they were free from migraine, asthma, epilepsy, or aggressive rages.

This does not occur in absolutely all PMS sufferers, however. There are a few—some 10 percent—who find that their symptoms continue throughout pregnancy: they develop marked weight gain, and also possibly raised blood pressure and protein in the urine, signs of preeclampsia. These women have an underdeveloped placenta, but they can still be helped with progesterone therapy throughout pregnancy. Controlled trials in the 1960s showed the benefits of giving progesterone to women with these symptoms during mid-pregnancy (see *Alison*, pages 260–261): the rate of preeclampsia was reduced from 10 percent in those receiving only symptomatic treatment to 3 percent among women receiving progesterone by injection or suppository.

THE EFFECTS OF PROGESTERONE DURING PREGNANCY

In the early sixties, reports were received that children whose mothers had been given progestogens during early pregnancy tended to have fetal abnormalities. This was especially true of female children, who showed evidence of masculinization of the genital organs. This was not surprising, because at that time the progestogens were all testosterone derivatives; but few doctors appreciated the differences between natural progesterone and the artificial progestogens. So the use of progesterone in pregnancy was generally stopped and has only recently been restarted with the introduction of in vitro fertilization, in which progesterone is essential for successful implantation. The progesterone given in treatment has exactly the same formula as the natural progesterone produced by the placenta and ovaries, so there are no side effects. It has usually been synthesized from yams and, more recently, from soybeans.

Starting in 1959, a twenty-year controlled study at the City of London Maternity Hospital was carried out on all children whose mothers received progesterone during pregnancy for the relief of excessive vomiting and other symptoms. The study showed that at the age of one, the progesterone children stood and walked earlier, but there was no difference in talking or teething; at nine to ten years, the progesterone children were noted to be above average in academic subjects—English, verbal reasoning, and arithmetic—but not in craft work or physical education. The progesterone children did better at school, graduating at sixteen and eighteen years; and finally, 32 percent went on to college, compared to only 6 percent of the controls (6 percent was also the national British and London average). The children who received progesterone early—before the sixteenth week of pregnancy—were those who benefited most (see Alison, pages 260–261).

WHAT TO EXPECT AFTER CHILDBIRTH

At birth, the placenta comes away from the womb, and suddenly, within twenty-four hours, the high level of progesterone in the mother's blood drops to nearly zero and her breasts start milk production, stimulated by another hormone, prolactin. Menstruation does not normally occur until after breast-feeding has stopped. Symptoms of PMS may suddenly occur out of the blue several days before the first menstruation after the baby's birth. After the euphoria of holding her baby in her arms, the majority of mothers experience days of unexpected tearfulness or "the blues." These are tears of emotion, not real depression, occurring during the first two weeks, and normally all is well thereafter.

In one new mother in ten, however, things may not go right after the birth. She may unexpectedly develop anxiety, agitation, insomnia, irritability, confusion, hallucinations, and tearfulness, and she may reject the baby or even harm her longed-for child. This is known as *postnatal depression*, which is better called postnatal illness (PNI), because depression is not necessarily present, nor is it the main symptom. Unfortunately, women who have had PMS are prone to develop postnatal illness, but the good news is that PNI can be prevented by receiving progesterone injections starting immediately after delivery and continuing for seven days, and then using progesterone suppositories (see *Pippa*, pages 261–262).

Women who have had postnatal depression once have around a 68 percent chance of having it again after another pregnancy, but trials of prophylactic progesterone worldwide have shown that it is possible to reduce this recurrence rate to 7 percent. (See the publications at the back of the book for details.)

MATERNAL BEHAVIOR AND POSTPARTUM ILLNESS

We are all familiar with TV documentaries showing examples of maternal behavior in animals—the mother bird feeding its young or the pig with numerous piglets suckling happily. Scientists have studied maternal behavior in laboratory animals, noting their effectiveness in keeping their newborns fed, cleaned, warm, and protected. Scientists know that maternal behavior develops naturally only when the female animal has been pregnant. In rats, mice, sheep, and monkeys, however, they have been able to show that maternal behavior can be artificially produced even in females that have never been pregnant. Virgin females are given a course of progesterone and estrogen, such as would normally be produced during a pregnancy, and placed near newborn young of the same species. The treated animals will then try to feed, clean, keep warm, and protect the young. This demonstrates that maternal behavior, or the maternal instinct, is hormonally influenced at least if not completely under hormonal control.

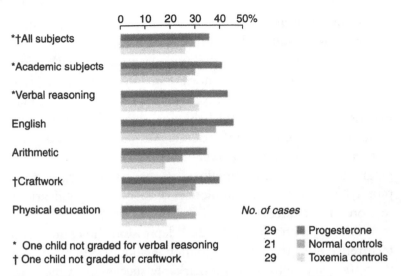

Figure 55   Above-average grades of seventy-nine children nine
to ten years old

More recently, scientists have been able to immunize virgin
female rats and mice so that they develop progesterone antibodies, or progesterone-receptor antibodies. These immunized animals take slightly longer than normal to conceive, but they have
a normal, full-term pregnancy and normal labor. However, if
after delivery they are moved in their cage a short distance from
the litter, the immunized animals will neglect their young: they
show no maternal behavior, they reject their young, and they
may even cannibalize them. On the other hand, control animals
moved a short distance from their young immediately after delivery will search for their young and either retrieve them or make
a new nest for them, while showing full maternal behavior.
Furthermore, if immunized animals with progesterone antibodies
are again mated, there is no delay in conception and again they
have a normal pregnancy and labor but again show loss of maternal behavior and reject their young or cannibalize them.

What the biologists call "maternal behavior" we would
call the "maternal instinct" and love that develop during pregnancy. Often, a pregnancy that was unplanned and unwanted

in the first few weeks becomes a much-wanted baby when delivered as a result of the hormones of pregnancy.

This exciting work is helping us understand the true nature of postnatal illness, a hormonal illness linked to progesterone. In severe cases of postnatal depression, women may experience loss of maternal behavior, reject their baby, and sometimes even commit infanticide. Also, if postnatal depression occurs once, it is very likely to be repeated in subsequent pregnancies. This also explains the success of progesterone prophylaxis given after completion of labor (see publications section for references).

After one attack of postnatal depression the chance of a recurrence after the next pregnancy is about 68 percent, but progesterone prophylaxis is remarkably successful in preventing it. If progesterone is given immediately after labor and continued for the next two months or until menstruation returns, the chance of a recurrence drops to between 7 percent and 10 percent. Such progesterone prevention is advised and should be organized during pregnancy for sufferers of severe PMS, for those who have a mother or sister who has experienced postnatal depression, and, most important of all, for those who have previously suffered from postnatal depression. The day may come when all women can receive treatment to prevent postnatal depression. Mothers can breast-feed while receiving progesterone; indeed, progesterone enhances lactation, which is an additional bonus.

28

Clinical Trials

Gradually there has been a change from anecdotal medicine to evidence-based medicine. Anecdotal medicine is now regarded as old-fashioned; it refers to the practice of studying individuals, listening to their symptoms, examining them, and noting and recording their responses to both immediate and long-term treatment. This is quite different from evidence-based medicine, which is based on a study of the results of double-blind, placebo-controlled trials.

There are many difficulties in clinical trials of PMS, in which there are over 150 different symptoms to be considered, symptoms varying in severity from very mild warnings of menstruation to life-threatening ones. For ethical reasons, patients are not allowed to enter clinical trials, which usually last six months, if they have ever been treated for their symptoms in a hospital, or have a history of violence, epilepsy, self-mutilation, or life-threatening behavior. Volunteers in clinical trials must be prepared to go without any medication, a rule that effectively prevents epileptics and asthmatics from enrolling. They must not use either hormonal contraception or an intrauterine device, and they cannot plan to be pregnant for the duration of the trials. Volunteers need to be conscientious and ready to complete a questionnaire regularly, often every day. So the call is for abnormally obsessive and introverted women, who will record daily, even on those days when they have a severe migraine, have experienced a bereavement, have taken an overnight holiday flight, or have attended an all-night party. One is tempted to ask whether these volunteers are normal, typical PMS sufferers. In short, volunteers are limited to a small number of women with such mild PMS that they are prepared to go without any other medication for six months. Suitable volunteers are difficult to find. Frequently, there have to be media calls for local volunteers. Another problem is the high number of women who initially enroll but then drop out. How should the dropouts be counted? Why did they drop out? Did they stop because of the daily chore of completing the questionnaires? Because they developed side effects? Because they went on vacation? Because they got worse or got better?

All trials on PMS have shown a high placebo response, which means that during the first month of having either effective medication or a placebo, all patients in the study improve. The reason is unknown. There have been many suggestions but no consensus of opinion. In 1982, three London gynecologists, A. L. Magos, M. Brincot, and J.W.W. Studd, studied the effect of implants on sixty-eight women with PMS. They either gave a normal estrogen implant, or just anesthetized the skin, cut the usual half-inch incision, and sewed up the skin without inserting a pellet of estrogen. They reported that after the first month 94 percent of those who had received a fake implant improved. Unfortunately, the placebo effect did not last long, and by the next month their symptoms were as bad as ever. Taking into account this high placebo effect, statisticians calculate that any successful PMS trial will need at least 120 women to complete a six-month study.

In Britain now, clinical trials are carefully controlled and permission must be granted from the ethics committee of the hospital or area health committee before commencing work. The ethics committee must see the protocol showing precisely which patients are to be included and excluded, and the written information to be given to the volunteers about the details of the trial, together with a copy of the consent form that all women will be asked to sign before entering the trials. No more mock operations will be allowed without the patient's knowledge and consent.

The following are the special problems associated with PMS trials of progesterone.

Prolems with PMS Trials

- The precise definition of PMS must be followed, with absence of symptoms in the postmenstruum.
- There is a high dropout rate.
- There is a high placebo response.
- Trials take a long time; at least six months of daily recording is needed.
- A high number of volunteers is required
- There are150 possible symptoms, both psychological and physical.
- Trials are limited to mild cases for ethical reasons.
- Participating women must have regular menstrual cycles.
- The women must not be using hormonal contraception or IUDs.
- Participants cannot plan to be pregnant within six months.
- Participants may take no medicine for the duration of the trials, neither prescribed nor over-the-counter medication.

Trials usually last six months, with the first two months devoted to daily recording of symptoms and the presence or absence of menstruation. If the two months of recording confirm the precise definition of PMS, the volunteer will then be allocated either to a treatment group having two cycles of active medication followed by two cycles of placebo medication or to the group having two placebo-treated cycles followed by two cycles with active medication. The active medication and the

placebo medication will look similar and will have been prepared by the drug firm, so that even the doctors monitoring
the trials will not know to which group a patient belongs.

Up to now there has been only one successful trial,
authored by Dr. Pat Magill and reported in the *British Journal
of General Practitioners*. It was a multicentered general-practi-
tioner trial using a dose of suppositories 400 mg twice daily
from ovulation to menstruation. Previous trials had used
smaller doses of progesterone suppositories by practitioners,
who did not appreciate that estrogen is measured in picograms
and progesterone in nanograms (see pages 70–72).

It will be noted that even in the successful Magill trial,
no consideration was given to the diet of the volunteers nor to
the incidence of smoking, both of which reduce the effectiveness of progesterone receptors. Including these two factors
would make clinical trials even more difficult, with eating
habits controlled every single day for six months, which would
inevitably include Christmas or other holidays.

There are different problems associated with double-
blind, placebo-controlled trials into progesterone prevention
of a recurrence of postnatal depression. Too many women have
received treatment, or know someone who received treatment
since the first report in the *Practitioner* in 1985. Today, if a volunteer who has once suffered from postnatal depression agrees
to participate in clinical trials of progesterone prevention, she
knows there is only a 50 percent chance of effective treatment;
whereas if she refuses, there is more than a 90 percent chance
of preventing a recurrence. The trials will need to be conducted in a country that does not routinely use progesterone to
prevent the recurrence of postnatal depression.

29

※

How Are They Now?

PMS is a chronic disease. Although there will be times during the menstruating years when symptoms are milder or absent, PMS will always be lurking in the background, ready to come back at times of stress or with other illnesses or accidents, night work, jet lag, excess alcohol intake, or a strict weight-reducing diet. Progesterone will not always be required, but the need for the frequent Three-Hourly Starch Diet remains. After menopause, progesterone is not required for reproduction, but it is still valuable for preventing osteoporosis, for serotonin metabolism, and for respiration, blood vessels, skin, and hair. Some women benefit from progesterone even in the postmenopausal years.

My work on PMS started in 1948, so I have been able to follow up on several thousands of patients for many years. This chapter is designed to give some idea of the variety of PMS and the subsequent stories of a few women mentioned (and cross-referenced) in the text. All names are fictitious, and examples that might be known to the media have been excluded except for the first two women, who have written their own accounts.

A book by Nicola Owen, *Nicola: A Second Chance to Live*, published in 1992 by Bantam, relates how at puberty Nicola became a compulsive eater, suffered violent mood swings, engaged in self-mutilation, and was described as a "hysterical psychopath" when in prison for arson (*Nicola's* early story can be found on pages 174–176). She made legal history as the first case in which PMS was used as a defense for a charge of arson. Nicola is Case 2 in my paper "Cyclical Criminal Acts in Premenstrual Syndrome" in *The Lancet* (1980), and the search for her evidence is described on pages 110–113 of my book *Premenstrual Syndrome Goes to Court*. Once Nicola's PMS was diagnosed and treated, her whole life changed. Today she is charming, married with one child, and a highly effective business executive.

Anna Reynolds (page 178) hid her pregnancy from her mother, gave up the baby for adoption, and later, in an uncontrollable PMS rage, murdered her mother. She was serving a life sentence when evidence of PMS emerged and she was freed on probation. An account of her defense is on pages 112–113 of *Premenstrual Syndrome Goes to Court*. Her tragic story is told in her book *Tightrope* (Sidgwick & Jackson) and another book, *Insanity*. She is now a successful playwright, and critics have been most enthusiastic about her three plays currently showing in London.

Dina (page 2), who was thirty-one at the time, operated a hair salon with her husband and had a five-year-old daughter when I first met her in 1961. She had been in good health until her pregnancy, which was complicated by severe preeclampsia and excessive weight gain. Since then she had suffered from marked bloating, headaches, and wild tempers premenstrually, but she still had a sense of humor and told endless jokes on her good days after menstruation. Once, when she caught her daughter cutting up an expensive satin quilt, she threw her across the bed in a fit of temper. On another occasion, Dina smashed up her daughter's prized guitar. Dina changed when progesterone treatment was started, and she never looked back. Many times an effort was made—unsuccessfully—to reduce the progesterone, and now, after more than thirty years, she still needs it. She has since been widowed and lives alone with three dogs. Her daughter now has an M.S. degree and is a freelance lecturer in horticulture and curator of one of our city's botanical gardens.

Margaret (page 61) was twenty-seven years old, with two daughters, aged four and one, when first treated in 1968 for premenstrual epileptic attacks. During these attacks, she would be unconscious for about three hours, so could not be left alone to look after her children, who were put into foster care. She had been in the metabolic unit of a mental hospital for two months, but the doctors·had failed to find a solution. Progesterone therapy was effective, and after twelve months she was able to look after the children again. When she regained her health, she took up psychiatric nursing, winning several prizes on the way. Over the years she has worked in various nursing positions and now is the head of a home for disturbed adults. Needless to say, she is among the best diagnosticians of PMS and ensures that many of her patients receive appropriate PMS treatment. Her children are both married with children of their own, and they do not appear to have suffered unduly from their mother's absence in their early life.

Sara (page 60) was an eighteen-year-old student whose education had been blighted by severe asthma, requiring more than twenty hospital admissions into intensive care, until an alert night nurse recognized the pattern of premenstrual episodes. I first saw her in 1980 when she was hoping to enter medical school, but she was in the hospital at the time of exams. She responded to progesterone therapy, completed a law degree, and became a successful commercial lawyer. She had a good personal relationship for seven years, but when that ended in 1992 she had another return of severe asthma, again requiring intensive care. She was referred to a gynecologist who prescribed estrogen patches. After her third day on estrogen patches she again had a life-threatening attack. The hospital director faxed for an urgent appointment, and progesterone was restarted. Her Christmas card in 1996 advised me that she had enjoyed a year without seeing the inside of a hospital. Then, unusually, her problem changed to estrogen dominance, and she benefited from a total hysterectomy. She now enjoys good health, so good that she is pursuing a biochemistry degree as a mature student, intending to study medicine. I wish her well and believe she will be a wonderful, understanding doctor.

Laura (page 61), a forty-three-year-old part-time secretary, was first seen for PMS in 1979. She had had her first epileptic seizure at nineteen and had typical EEG changes, so she had been on anticonvulsants ever since. It was recognized that the seizures only occurred premenstrually. Her husband noticed that the attacks were preceded by irritability, headaches, getting "het up," and "thinking too far ahead." Since 1972 she had been having depot progestogen (Depo-Provera)injections, which had not helped. She indicated that she ate her three daily meals five hours apart and went fourteen hours overnight without food. Even in those days, she was advised to eat starchy food frequently and was started on progesterone. The attack described on page 61 was her last until February 1994, when she phoned to tell me she had had an unexpected attack and was being investigated at the hospital.

Laura had two further sudden losses of consciousness in March and April 1994, which were thoroughly investigated with the most modern neurological techniques, but no abnormality was discovered. At sixty-two years she was leading a full social life with her retired husband, enjoying golf several times a week and traveling. However, when we investigated the full circumstances of each of the three attacks, a common factor emerged. Each attack occurred following a special occasion when she had enjoyed a special dinner with liberal alcohol. The next day she had awakened with a headache and missed breakfast, and the attacks occurred while she was active in the late morning, on one occasion on the golf course. When this connection was made, she vowed never to miss breakfast again, and she would be wise to be moderate with alcohol in the future.

Jessica (pages 111–112) had her first period in August 1982 at the age of thirteen. Her menstruation was not regular; in fact, she only had two periods in the next six months. Nevertheless, for two weeks each month she became severely depressed and anxious, with fears of dying. Twice she had a short hospital admission and, being unable to attend school, had a home tutor for two hours daily. Her parents recognized the deterioration that occurred at monthly intervals and so Jessica had almost daily hormone estimations taken for two months. I then saw her, and even before the results of blood tests were known she was started on progesterone. She had a good response to it—so good that she was able to return to school and finish her education. Jessica became a licensed hairdresser and remained free from depression until 1993. With her wedding pending she went on a drastic weight-reducing diet and relapsed, with such severe irritability, depression, anxiety, and claustrophobia that she canceled the wedding. When she resumed the Three-Hourly Starch Diet and progesterone, her premenstrual symptoms disappeared, and she married six months later. Her parents divorced, and later she divorced. In 1998, because of a large weight gain, she went on another rigid weight-reducing diet, and again relapsed, this time ending in a psychiatric hospital.

Loretta (page 149) was married to a doctor and worked as her husband's receptionist. She had two children, one of whom is now also a doctor. She changed from experiencing unexpected explosive moods to being calm and loving once her problem was treated. She continued with progesterone until she was sixty, and then gradually reduced the dose and stopped. She was widowed in 1998, and is now living alone and enjoying her two children and three grandchildren.

Julia (page 172), a thirty-three-year-old housewife, was charged with murder after an alcoholic binge during which she stabbed a friend. She had had four children by three different men. The social services were already aware that she would become violent premenstrually, but since the children were being cared for by different agencies, no one recognized the immensity of Julia's problem or made any attempt to arrange treatment for her or inform her general practitioner. The elder girl—twelve years old—had been in trouble at school and her parents were sent for twice. On both occasions, Julia was within a day of starting menstruation. The second child was a boy of nine, whose behavior was always good. Her third child was a boy of seven who was in a school for disturbed children. The school kept a record of the days on which the children became unruly, and it was from this record that it was noted that this boy's riotous behavior always occurred during Julia's premenstruum. The youngest child, aged four, was attending an enuretic clinic at the local hospital; his bedwetting was recorded daily and was also found to occur during Julia's premenstruum. Julia was released on bail, and when I first saw her she had smashed up the house during her previous premenstruum. The welfare officer who attended the consultation was able to confirm the damage Julia had done to an end table and a table lamp. The difference in her behavior once she was on a good diet and started on progesterone therapy was remarkable. She was freed on probation, which has now ended, and all her children are well behaved with good school reports. She has changed her last name and started a new life.

Anne (pages 176–177) was nineteen years old at our first meeting in 1979. After her release from prison, she continued to attend the Premenstrual Clinic at University College Hospital—a journey of about one hundred miles from her home—at intervals of three and six months. Before her marriage, I met her future husband and discussed with him Anne's diagnosis of PMS and the importance of continuing the Three-Hourly Starch Diet and progesterone treatment. She was supervised during her pregnancy and received progesterone prophylaxis immediately after delivery to ensure that she did not develop postnatal depression. Her son was born in 1988, and Anne saw me once when he was six weeks old and fully breastfed. However, the long journey to London proved too much for her, so her general practitioner took over her supervision.

One day when she was out with her husband at a garage sale they bought a book on PMS that advocated 100 mg of pyridoxine (vitamin B-6) daily. This sounded much better than and a relief from frequent injections, so her doctor agreed and changed the prescription in October 1992. Anne's mother was the first to notice that Anne seemed to lack energy and occasionally became confused. Anne and her husband were having financial problems, so to help the family budget Anne stopped eating breakfast, dulling her hunger by smoking instead.

In February 1993, quite unexpectedly, Anne was arrested for making fake bomb threats. She resisted arrest and was charged with injuring a police officer. Full particulars are described in Case 3 in "Cyclical Criminal Acts in Premenstrual Syndrome" in *The Lancet* (1980). In the police station she was immediately given progesterone injections, and her husband soon noticed an improvement in her condition. It was extraordinary that she should revert to the same type of criminal behavior after an interval of twelve years during which her behavior had been exemplary.

Jean (page 179) had suffered from PMS since puberty, as was noted in her medical file, until she was advised at age seventeen to stop taking the Pill because of migraines and hypertension. She had a teenage pregnancy and gave the baby up for adoption. She was very healthy during her second, planned, pregnancy—in fact, her husband described it as a "radiant happiness."

She had severe postnatal illness, during which she drowned her baby and then tried to stab herself in the abdomen, slashed her wrists, and took an overdose. On recovering consciousness in the hospital, she was devastated by the loss of her baby and was allowed home on bail to be comforted by her husband and parents. When I first saw Jean, she had begun menstruation and had noticeable PMS. She was started on progesterone—injections initially and suppositories later. Although she pleaded guilty to infanticide, she was freed on probation. The director and staff of the local social services were so impressed by her improvement that they asked me to give a public lecture on PMS.

Jean had left school early without receiving a degree, so she returned as a reentry student, majoring in math and biology.

She had another planned pregnancy, during which she received progesterone. She also received prophylactic progesterone against postnatal depression. All went well, and her healthy daughter was taken off the At-Risk Register when she was six months old. Jean is well adjusted, is living in the present, and has realistic plans for the future.

Angela (page 185) had an ovarian cyst removed when she was sixteen, suffered from postnatal depression after the birth of her third child, and had a hysterectomy with removal of both ovaries in 1974. She was given progesterone suppositories and after the first month she was reported to be calmer, with no more days in bed. Over the next few years she was free from symptoms, and she was discharged from the PMS Clinic in 1978. She was active, leading a full life, and teaching squash. Suddenly she deteriorated at Christmas 1982 when within a few days my notes record that she suddenly became "het up—disinterested—could not concentrate—slowed, but no tears." She improved within three days of being treated with progesterone, and this was stopped after two months. Surprisingly, her condition again deteriorated two days after Christmas in 1985 and 1990, and on both occasions benefited from progesterone. Whether it was due to the tensions of the preparations for Christmas, the extra champagne and chocolates, or the stress of the family gatherings is unknown, but she has had prophylactic progesterone in the last two Decembers with apparent success. She remains an enigma.

Alison (page 244) was discussed in the British Medical Journal in August 1957 in my paper "Toxemia of Pregnancy Treated with Progesterone During the Symptomatic Stage." The paper discussed how when progesterone is given for the relief of pregnancy symptoms, usually "treatment can be discontinued after the fourth of fifth month, but where necessary, treatment is maintained throughout pregnancy." Alison is an example of a woman who needed progesterone from the sixth week of pregnancy until labor, at thirty-four weeks. She was thirty-one years old, working in the garment industry, and had

had two previous miscarriages. She suffered from backaches, headaches, and exhaustion. These were eased with progesterone, taken daily or on alternate days. In those days progesterone could only be given intramuscularly. Attempts were made at twelve, sixteen, and twenty-two weeks of pregnancy to stop the progesterone, but her symptoms immediately returned.

Alison had an easy labor and gave birth to fraternal twins, who weighed 4 lb. 1 oz and 3 lb. 13 oz. Following the pregnancy, she had no postnatal depression or PMS and had no further need for progesterone. At the age of thirty-eight she became hypothyroid and benefited from thyroid replacement, but over the years she has again occasionally become hyperthyroid. She had an easy menopause and enjoyed good health until 1990, when she was found to have severe osteoporosis, with only 76 percent of bone mineral density compared to normal women of her age and height. She had the typical risk factors of a family history (a sister with osteoporosis), lifelong avoidance of dairy products, lifelong weight maintenance below ideal weight, and thyroid medication. Fortunately, with ethidronate and progesterone treatment, her joint pains eased and her bone mineral density rose to 83 percent in the next three years. Unfortunately, she fractured her hip in 1997.

Alison's twins (page 245) were included in the twenty-year follow-up of children whose mothers received progesterone while pregnant, first reported in 1976 in the *British Journal of Psychiatry*. They developed early, standing at seven months and walking at nine months, and they made excellent progress in school, both winning scholarships to a fee-paying school noted for its high academic standards, both going on to college and gaining good degrees. One is a successful accountant, married, with a son and daughter, and the other a successful physicist, with one son.

Pippa (page 246), a radiographer, was twenty-five years old and her baby was nine months when she was first seen in 1983. She had no previous psychiatric symptoms or illnesses, and she described her pregnancy as "great—bloomed."

However, following a normal labor and birth, she experienced a personality change. By the third day after giving birth, she was hostile to her husband, screaming, dissatisfied, delusional, and having hallucinations. She was admitted to a mother and baby unit, where she became violent with the nurses. For safety precautions, her baby was removed from her care for a few days. Pippa later described the treatment during her five-week hospital stay as "barbaric." Interestingly, Pippa had a similar family history: her mother had also suffered delusions after Pippa's birth and her sister had suffered postnatal depression.

Because of her terrifying experience, Pippa was anxious to be sterilized to ensure that she would never have to go through that hell again. She and her husband considered adopting if they wished to have any more children. At our first meeting, I discussed the hormonal cause of postnatal psychosis and its successful prevention with progesterone. In 1985, Pippa had the courage to become pregnant again and underwent prophylactic progesterone. On the third day, two hours before her next injection, she felt "strange," so she had an early injection and immediately felt "wonderful." Subsequently, in addition to her daily injections she had suppositories for a few days. She was able to enjoy those first few months of her baby's life and breast-fed her successfully. I met Pippa quite accidentally in 1994 at a health workers' conference in London. She presented a paper, "The Effect of Postnatal Depression on the Family." An elegant and first-class speaker, she spoke from her heart. She is now a successful lecturer on radiation safety, traveling widely to Europe and beyond. Her message at the conference was that there was life after postnatal depression and that postnatal depression can be prevented. She proudly showed a photograph of her two healthy, happy daughters.

The diversity of these thumbnail sketches merely serves to emphasize that we women are all different, and medically each one of us needs to be considered individually. There remains considerable work before our personal hormonal changes can be fully understood.

30

⁂

A Fairer Future

This book is written with the aim of spreading the news that the once-a-month miseries of countless women can be, and are being, successfully treated and relieved. It is also written to help men understand and appreciate the menstrual problems of women and become partners in helping them through their difficult days. That you are reading this book brings hope that the aim will be achieved.

Menstrual problems are widespread and often incapacitating. All classes, all ages, and both sexes feel their effects. Currently it is possible to eliminate dysmenorrhea, PMS, and menopausal problems by giving hormone therapy; but although treatment is possible, it is not yet universal. Menopausal clinics are now well established, so that gynecological help is available nationwide for the relief of symptoms related to the change of life. The recognition of PMS is not as widespread, although there have been many encouraging developments since the first edition of this book.

In 1983, Mrs. Lindsay Burton Leckie and Mrs. Pat Cannon, who had both suffered from PMS and benefited from progesterone therapy, founded the National PMS Society, a nonprofit, all-volunteer educational and support network consisting of ninety-one affiliated groups throughout the United

States. Their goals were to educate the medical and lay communities in the identification and treatment of PMS, to promote an awareness of the existence of PMS among the general public, and to assist women by offering emotional support and updated information. Though the society is now defunct, much of its good work is being carried on by independent groups, which offer literature and newsletters on PMS. Other activities include walk-in counseling, telephone hotlines, public meetings, workshops and seminars, and fundraising for PMS research. For a list of clinics and support and information groups, see the Appendix on page 285.

A SPECIALTY OF THE FAMILY PHYSICIAN

PMS should really be a specialty of family practice, and it should be mastered by every family physician. Someday, every generalist and consultant will be able to diagnose, treat, and manage all cases of PMS that come within their orbit. The long-term follow-up of a chronic disease such as PMS is best done by the physician of continuing care, rather than in hospitals, with their ever-changing junior staff and their need to discharge patients as soon as possible to make way for new ones. At present, however, this goal is a long way off.

Gynecologists tend to be satisfied with normality on full examination, as discussed in chapter 8. Endocrinologists feel they have more serious diseases to occupy their time and rarely trouble themselves with disturbances of the menstrual hormones, especially at a time when there are not enough useful hormonal estimations to confirm a diagnosis and determine the dosage of hormones needed. Psychiatrists do occasionally recognize the syndrome and prescribe antidepressants or tranquilizers, but they may next see the patient during her symptom-free postmenstruum and decide she no longer needs care. Neurologists will investigate all cases of epilepsy and migraines to ensure that no lesion is present, and discharge the patient. The chest doctor treats the asthma, the rhinologist treats the allergic rhinitis, the orthopedic surgeon and rheumatologist treat the backache and painful joints, the dermatologist treats the herpes and neurodermatitis, and so on. But even if all these menstrually related symptoms are known to the specialists, the overall diagnosis may easily be ignored.

For a very short time only the University of Oklahoma led the world in having a department of Premenstrual Syndrome, with a multidisciplinary staff working together to bring relief to PMS sufferers. Their responsibility included conducting clinics for the diagnosis and treatment of PMS, teaching medical students and residents, and organizing research aimed at helping women worldwide.

WHY IS PMS SO BADLY TREATED?

Having read so far in the book, you may be wondering, "If progesterone results in such successful relief, why aren't more doctors using it, and why aren't they telling us about the Three-Hourly Starch Diet?" "Why do some doctors prefer to use a less successful drug that only brings partial relief to a few patients with mild symptoms, rather than follow a regime that brings complete relief to most patients with mild, moderate, or severe symptoms?"

There is no simple answer to these perfectly reasonable questions. Some answers are contained in earlier chapters, and there are other possible reasons, which come under three broad headings:

1. Doctors are essentially conservative.

2. Commercial considerations play a large role.

3. There is a lack of consultancy and treatment facilities for PMS.

Whereas medicine was once an art, recognizing that we are all individuals and different, today medicine is a science, one that considers us all to be the same. This means that the double-blind placebo-controlled trial is the god, and there is no longer a place for anecdotal medicine. Yet the origin of evidence-based medicine lay in anecdotal observations, such as that rubella in early pregnancy may result in fetal deformity, as does thalidomide; both penicillin and the vaccination for smallpox resulted from anecdotal evidence. Doctors in those days did not wait for the evidence of double-blind controlled trials. Incidentally, it may interest many readers to know that insulin for diabetes has never been subjected to double-blind controlled trials, but we know it works. Nor has in vitro fertilization ever been subjected to controlled trials, but we know it also works.

Very few doctors practicing today have had any real training in diagnosing or treating what we know to be the world's most common disease, PMS. Doctors are wholly responsible for the diagnosis and treatment of their patients. They have the right and the responsibility to protect their patients and themselves, so they are naturally reluctant to use treatments that are new or not yet fully established as safe and effective. However, doctors are also responsible for continually increasing their medical knowledge. In Britain it is estimated that an average general practitioner has about fifty women in his or her practice needing treatment for PMS. Another factor is that doctors receive little or no training in nutrition, and rarely if ever ask a patient for a detailed account of her usual or previous day's diet. Some may say that there is no time to take a dietary history, but a nurse or assistant could easily do this.

One cannot ignore commercial pressures in today's world. The formula of progesterone was discovered in 1934 and thus is not protected by a patent, so no drug manufacturer will benefit financially from marketing it. The costs of clinical trials and of gathering the necessary evidence to convince the Food and Drug Administration of the effectiveness of progesterone in the treatment of PMS are high. If any manufacturer succeeds in getting a license, there is no guarantee of profit, because any other manufacturer could use the expensively obtained evidence to produce a similar product. Vitamins and minerals, on the other hand, are a good source of profit because they can be advertised to the general public and sold over the counter without a medical prescription and without the need to prove their effectiveness, which can be expensive. Unfortunately, vitamins and minerals offer no special benefit to women with PMS.

Family physicians who have patients with a condition that is hard to diagnose can send them to a specialist. But to whom can they send their cases of premenstrual asthma or premenstrual sinusitis, which have been confirmed by menstrual charts? Not to a gynecologist or endocrinologist or psychiatrist. Consulting specialists in the field of PMS just do not exist. This is where the real need is—for a new specialty of PMS. At present it is sometimes covered in England by the Well Woman Clinics, which busy themselves with family planning and menopause, but the specialists will need to update their knowledge, know the use of the menstrual chart, and recognize the problems of progesterone receptors and the need for the Three-Hourly Starch Diet.

HOPE FOR THE FUTURE

In 1986 the Dalton Society, an international medical society of doctors, was founded with the object of furthering knowledge of and research into PMS. The society has held conferences in Los Angeles, Chicago, Tulsa, Oklahoma City, San Francisco, London, and Perth, attended by doctors from around the world, where research papers were read and discussions held on improvements in treatment and a better understanding of the causes of PMS. The research papers read at a meeting of the Royal Society of Medicine in London in 1992 entitled "Progesterone—Its Many Clinical Uses" were published in the *British Journal of Family Planning.* There are also "friends of the society," who, although not in the medical field, contribute funds and energy to the alleviation of the problems brought on by PMS, surely a worthwhile charity deserving of generous support.

PREMENSTRUAL SYNDROME CLINICS

In Britain in 1985 the National Commission for Women passed a resolution calling the government's attention to the need for greater undergraduate and postgraduate education on PMS, and the need for training teachers, social workers, police, and lawyers about this subject. It is to be regretted that subsequent governments have not given consideration to this issue.

If PMS clinics are to be established, the skilled generalist director needs to have on his or her staff, among others, a nurse to teach menstrual charting, a psychiatrist, a gynecologist, a nutritionist, and a counselor. Only a generalist deals with the whole range of PMS symptoms and has an idea of the effect on the family. There remains a need for medical courses specialized in diagnosing, treating, and updating our knowledge about progesterone and progesterone receptors. Medical students should be made more familiar with the subject during their undergraduate training. There is also a need to learn the art of scheduling important events during the alert postmenstruum, understanding the methods and the risks, knowing how to help women best utilize their peak postmenstrual days, and learning to recognize those women with dysmenorrhea and PMS, who need urgent treatment.

The need for greater public education and awareness is obvious. And a very real opportunity exists for the media to educate a public that welcomes human-interest stories and news of medical possibilities. The media should be particularly good at emphasizing the need to chart the days of menstruation and problem times, and also teaching the reason for and effectiveness of the Three-Hourly Starch Diet. We must remember, however, that doctors do not like to be told by the press what treatment they should give their patients. Education on menstruation is already included in the curriculum of British high schools. This should help both the women and the men of tomorrow to have a greater understanding of the problems that exist and the solutions that are available.

Menstrual problems are estimated to cost American industry 8 percent of total wages paid. Surely it would be better to invest a fraction of that amount in menstrual clinics and training programs for doctors, in order to prevent the loss of all those working hours.

School and university examination boards in many countries have appreciated the effects of the menstrual handicap and now take PMS into consideration when designating the annual academic requirements, by adjusting schedules and offering alternative examination dates where possible, especially for laboratories and oral examinations.

A better understanding of the relationship between PMS and social and domestic violence would enable premenstrual baby battering and child abuse to be correctly diagnosed, understood, and treated. This could reduce the problems of children being separated from their parents and taken into foster care, and criminal proceedings against the mother.

Confronted with all these issues, one might think it would be best to abolish menstruation altogether at those times when conception is not required. As discussed, this can be done by the prolonged administration of progestogens, but it is not yet completely safe. Initially, there tends to be occasional breakthrough bleeding, and then, after a year or two, there is a subtle change in the woman's personality: she becomes harder and more efficient, with a high risk of osteoporosis and with a loss of sex interest. Is the price worth it? Many women eagerly hope that removal of the womb will solve the problem of menstruation, but as discussed in chapter 20, removal of the womb often upsets the hormonal pathway, and the end result may be worse than the preoperative condition.

In the last century, essayist John Ruskin reminded us that "the true wealth of the Nation was running to waste" because most children had no education. The same applies today in respect to the lack of education and understanding about PMS. Discussion of menstruation and menstrual problems should be as open and unrestricted as the discussion of sex, and information about menstruation should be available to all.

To quote Henry David Thoreau,

If you have built
Castles in the air,
Your work need
Not be lost;
There is where they
Should be.
Now put foundations under them.
Let us get down to work.

Glossary

Abortion—death of the fetus

Adolescence—the years between childhood and maturity

Adrenal glands—two glands situated above the kidneys and responsible for producing numerous hormones

Adrenaline—one of the hormones produced by the adrenal glands

Amenorrhea—absence of menstruation

Amnesia—loss of memory

Analgesic—drug taken to relieve pain

Anovular—without ovulation

Anorexia—loss of appetite

Antenatal—before childbirth

Antidepressant—drug to remove depression

Bromocriptine—drug that lowers the prolactin level

Candida—yeast infection

Cervical smear—test for the diagnosis of cancer of the neck of the womb

Cervix—neck of the womb

Climacteric—change of life

Conception—fertilization of the ovum

Corticosteroids—hormones produced in the cortex of the adrenal glands

Cystitis—inflammation of the urinary bladder

Diuretics—drugs capable of increasing the amount of urine passed

Dysmenorrhea—pain with periods

271

Embryo—developing ovum up to the end of the eighth week after conception

Endocrine gland—organ releasing hormones into the blood to act on distant cells

Endocrinologist—one who studies the effects of the endocrine glands

Endometrium—inner lining of the womb

Estrogen—hormone released by the ovary

Fallopian tubes—two tubes leading from the ovaries to the womb along which the egg cells pass

Fetus—developing human from three months to birth

Follicle-stimulating hormone (FSH)—hormone produced by the pituitary acting on the ovary to ripen the follicles and produce estrogen

Glaucoma—disease of the eye characterized by raised pressure in the eyeball

Glucose—a form of sugar found in the blood

Gonadotrophin—hormone produced by the pituitary acting on the gonads, either testes or ovary

Gynecology—study of the diseases of women

Hemorrhage—loss of blood, bleeding

Homicide—killing a human

Hormones—chemicals produced by the glands that have an action at a distant site

Hyperglycemia—raised blood sugar

Hypoglycemia—lowered blood sugar

Hypothalamus—specialized part of the brain concerned with control of body functions

Hysterectomy—surgical removal of the womb

Implant—pellets of drugs inserted into the tissues

Intermenstruum—part of the menstrual cycle not covered by the premenstruum or menstruation, usually Days 5 to 24

Infanticide—killing an infant

Insulin—hormone produced in the pancreas involved in glucose metabolism

Intrauterine device—small contraceptive device inserted into the womb

Labor—birthing of a baby

Lactation—breast-feeding

Lethargy—excessive tiredness

Libido—sex drive

Luteinizing hormone—hormone produced by the pituitary that causes ovulation and the production of progesterone

Mastitis—breast pain

Menarche—first menstruation

Menopause—last menstruation marking the end of the child-bearing years

Menstrual clock—specialized portion of the hypothalamus responsible for the cyclical timing of menstruation

Menstrual cycle—time from the first day of menstruation until the first day of the next menstruation

Menstrual loss—bleeding at menstruation

Menstruation—monthly bleeding from the vagina in women of childbearing age

Metabolism—building up and breaking down of chemicals in the body

Migraine—severe form of headache

Molecule—the smallest particle that contains the properties of that substance

Nucleus—the powerhouse in the center of every living cell

Nymphomania—excessive sex drive in women

Obese—excessively overweight

Ovary—reproductive organ containing egg cells

Ovulation—release of an egg cell from an ovary

Ovum—egg cell

Paramenstruum—premenstruum and menstruation

Pituitary—gland situated at the base of the brain and controlling many other glands

Placebo—inactive or inert substance with no curative value

Placenta—organ that develops within the womb, responsible for feeding the fetus and for the production of the hormones of pregnancy

Postmenstruum—the days immediately after menstruation

Postnatal—after childbirth

Potassium—mineral present in blood and cells of the body

Premenstruum—the days immediately prior to menstruation

Preovulatory—the days immediately before ovulation

Progesterone—hormone produced by the ovaries and adrenals, and by the placenta during pregnancy

Progestogen—synthetic drug, once thought to be a substitute for natural progesterone, used for contraception

Prolactin—hormone produced by the pituitary gland

Puerperium—time after childbirth

Pyridoxine—vitamin B-6

Receptor—compound capable of transporting chemicals within cells

Respiration—breathing

Rhinitis—hay fever

Salpingo-oophorectomy—surgical removal of the fallopian tubes and ovaries

Serotonin—chemical involved in brain metabolism

Sodium—mineral present in the blood and cells of the body

Spasmodic—coming in spasms

Sterilization—operation to permanently prevent conception

Synchrony—occurring at the same time

Syndrome—collection of symptoms that commonly occur together

Testosterone—male hormone

Therapy—treatment

Thrombosis—blood clot

Trauma—injury

Urethritis—inflammation of the urethra

Urology—study of the kidneys

Uterus—womb

Vagina—passage leading from the exterior of the female body to the mouth of the womb

Vaginitis—inflammation of the vagina

Vertigo—giddiness

Other Publications by the Author

BOOKS

1964: *The Premenstrual Syndrome*. William Heinemann Medical Books, London. (Translated into Spanish.)

1969: *The Menstrual Cycle*. Penguin Books, Harmondsworth, London; Pantheon Books, Random House, New York. (Translated into Spanish, Portuguese, French, Dutch, German, Swedish, Norwegian, and Danish.)

1977: *The Premenstrual Syndrome and Progesterone Therapy*. William Heinemann Medical Books, London; Year Book Medical Publishers, Chicago.

1978: *Once a Month*. Fontana Paperbacks, London; Hunter House, California, U.S.A. (Translated into Dutch.)

1980: *Depression After Childbirth*. Oxford University Press, Oxford. (Translated into Dutch, German, and Japanese.) Revised 2d edition, January 1989.

1984: *The Premenstrual Syndrome and Progesterone Therapy*. William Heinemann Medical Books, London; Year Book Medical Publishers, Chicago. Revised 2d edition.

1987: *Once a Month*. Fontana Paperbacks, London; Hunter House, California, U.S.A. Revised 3d edition. (Translated into Japanese.)

1990: *Once a Month*. Hunter House, California, U.S.A. Revised 4th edition.

1990: *Premenstrual Syndrome Illustrated*. Peter Andrew Publishing Co., Worcestershire, U.K.

1990: *Premenstrual Syndrome Goes to Court*. Peter Andrew Publishing Co., Worcestershire, U.K.

1994: *PMS—The Essential Guide to Treatment Options*. Dr. Katharina Dalton and David Holton. Thorsons, London, U.K.

1996: *Depression After Childbirth*, 3rd Edition. Oxford University Press, Oxford. (Translated into Japanese.)

1999: *Premenstrual Syndrome Goes to Court*. Peter Andrew Publishing Co., Worcestershire, U.K. (Translated into Japanese)

ORIGINAL PAPERS

9 May 1953: "The premenstrual syndrome." *British Medical Journal*, vol. 1, p. 1007. Joint authorship with Raymond Greene.

6 November 1954: "The similarity of symptomatology of premenstrual syndrome and toxaemia of pregnancy and their response to progesterone." *British Medical Journal*, vol. 2, p. 1071. BMA Prize.

May 1955: "Discussion on the premenstrual syndrome." *Proceedings of the Royal Society of Medicine*, vol. 48, no. 5, pp. 337–347 (Section of General Practice pp. 5–15).

December 1955: "Progesterone in toxaemia of pregnancy." *Medical World*.

1957: "The influence of menstruation on health & disease." *Proceedings of the Royal Society of Medicine*, vol. 57, no. 4, pp. 18–20.

June 1957: "The aftermath of hysterectomy and oophorectomy." *Proceedings of the Royal Society of Medicine*, vol. 50, no. 6, pp. 415–418 (Section of General Practice, pp. 13–16).

17 August 1957: "Toxaemia of pregnancy treated with progesterone during the symptomatic stage." *British Medical Journal*, vol. 2, pp. 378–381.

17 January 1959: "Menstruation and acute psychiatric illnesses." *British Medical Journal*, vol. 1, pp. 148–149.

1959: "Menstrual disorders in general practice." *Journal of the College of General Practitioners*, vol. 2, p. 236.

12 December 1959: "Comparative trials of new oral progestogenic compounds in treatment of premenstrual syndrome." *British Medical Journal*, vol. 2, pp. 1307–1309.

23 January 1960: "Early symptoms of pre-eclamptic toxaemia." *The Lancet*, vol. 1, pp. 198–199.

30 January 1960: "Effect of menstruation on schoolgirls' weekly work." *British Medical Journal*, vol. 1, pp. 326–328.

12 November 1960: "Menstruation and accidents." *British Medical Journal*, vol. 2, pp. 1425–1426.

3 December 1960: "Schoolgirls' behaviour and menstruation." *British Medical Journal*, vol. 2, pp. 1647–1649.

30 December 1961: "Menstruation and crime." *British Medical Journal*, vol. 2, pp. 1752–1753.

June 1962: "Controlled trials in the prophylactic value of progesterone in the treatment of pre-eclamptic toxaemia." *Journal of Obstetrics and Gynaecology of the British Commonwealth*, vol. 69, no. 3, pp. 463–468.

July 1963: "The present position of progestational steroids in the treatment of premenstrual syndrome." *Medical Women's Federation Journal*, pp. 137–140.

1964: "Notes on the use of the menstrual chart." *Drug and Therapeutics Bulletin*.

October 1966: "The influence of mother's menstruation on her child." *Proceedings of the Royal Society of Medicine*, vol. 59, no. 10, pp. 1014–1016, (Section of General Practice with Section on Paediatrics). BMA Prize.

October 1967: "Influence of menstruation on glaucoma." *British Journal Of Ophthalmology*, vol. 51, no. 10, pp. 692–695. BMA Prize.

1968: "Ante-natal progesterone and intelligence." *British Journal of Psychiatry*, vol. 114, pp. 1377–1382.

December 1968: "Menstruation and examinations." *The Lancet*, vol. 1, pp. 1386–1388.

March 1970: "The importance of menstrual dates." *Update*, vol. 2, pp. 310–314.

4 April 1970: "Children's hospital admissions and mother's menstruation." *British Medical Journal*, vol. 2, pp. 27–28.

June 1971: "Prospective study into puerperal depression." *British Journal of Psychiatry*, vol. 118, no. 547, pp. 689–692.

December 1971: "Puerperal and premenstrual depression." *Proceedings of the Royal Society of Medicine*, vol. 64, no. 12, pp. 1249–1252 (Section of General Practice, pp. 43–44).

19 February 1972: "Ovulation symptoms and avoidance of conception." *The Lancet*, vol. 1, pp. 437–438.

1973: "Migraine in general practice." *Journal of the Royal College of General Practitioners*, vol. 23, pp. 97–106. Migraine Trust Prize Essay 1972.

January 1973: "Progesterone suppositories and pessaries in the treatment of menstrual migraine." *Headache*, vol. 12, no. 4, pp. 151–159.

June 1973: "The general practitioner and research." *The Practitioner*, vol. 210, pp. 784–788.

October 1973: "Influence of Menstruation." *Update*. pp. 833–839.

13 May 1974: "Premenstrual ankle edema in young girl." *Journal of American Medical Association*, vol. 228.

1975: "Postpubertal Effects of Prenatal Administration of Progesterone." Society for Endocrine Congress, Amsterdam.

April 1975: "Do it yourself." *British Migraine Association*, Migraine Newsletter.

May 1975: "Menses and the Psyche." *General Practitioner*, vol. 1, p. 20.

3 May 1975: "Paramenstrual Baby Battering." *British Medical Journal*, vol. 2.

August 1975: "The effect of progesterone on brain function." *Proceedings of the Acta Endocrin Congress*, Amsterdam.

1975: "Postpubertal effects of prenatal administration of progesterone." Society for Research in Child Development.

July 1975: "Premenstrual syndrome." *Update*, pp. 121–128.

October 1975: "Food intake prior to a migraine attack—study of 2313 spontaneous attacks." *Headache*, vol. 15, no. 3, pp. 188–193.

January 1976: "Migraine and oral contraceptives." *Headache*, vol. 15, no. 4, pp. 247–251.

March 1976: "The Curse of Eve." *Occupational Health*. p. 129.

20 November 1976: "Progesterone or Progestogens?" *British Medical Journal*.

1976: "Prenatal progesterone and educational attainments." *British Journal of Psychiatry*, vol. 129, pp. 438–442. The Charles Oliver Hawthorne BMA Prize Essay 1976.

April 1976: "A clinician's view." *Royal Society of Health Journal*.

April 1976: "Menstruation and sport." Chapter in *Sports Medicine*, 2d edition. J. P. R. Williams and P. N. Sperry, Eds. Edward Arnold, London.

1976: "Treatment of the premenstrual syndrome." *Journal of Pharmacotherapy*, pp. 51–55.

1976: "Bromocriptine and premenstrual syndrome." Chapter in *Pharmacological and clinical aspects of Bromocriptine*. R. I. Bayliss, P. Turner, and W. P. McClay, Eds. M.S.C. Consultants, London.

February 1977: "Premenstrual Syndrome: Its Effects on Family Life." *Journal of Maternal and Child Health*. p. 69.

19 December 1977: "Premenstrual syndrome with psychiatric symptoms." *Journal of the American Medical Association*, vol. 238, no. 25, p. 2729.

1977: "Premenstrual Tension and Driving." *Royal Society of Prevention of Accidents*.

11 August 1978: "Synthetic progestins vs. natural generic progesterone: Pharmacologic properties." *Journal of the American Medical Association*, vol. 240, no. 6.

12 August 1978: "Menarcheal age in the disabled." *British Medical Journal*, no. 2, p. 475. Co-authored with Maureen E. Dalton.

1979: "Intelligence and prenatal progesterone: A reappraisal." *Journal of the Royal Society of Medicine*, vol. 72, pp. 397–399.

November 1979: "Food intake before migraine attacks in children." *Journal of the Royal College of General Practitioners*, no. 29, pp. 662–665. Joint authorship with Maureen E. Dalton.

December 1979: "Intelligence and prenatal progesterone." *Journal of the Royal Society of Medicine*, vol. 72, p. 951.

26 September 1980: "Cyclic posthysterectomy symptoms." *Journal of the American Medicine Association*, vol. 244, no. 13, p. 1497.

15 November 1980: "Cyclical criminal acts in premenstrual syndrome." *The Lancet*, pp. 1070–1071.

1981: "The effect of progesterone and progestogens on the foetus." *Neuropharmacology*.

1981: "Violence and the premenstrual syndrome." *Journal of Police Surgeons*, Great Britain.

1981: "The Menopause and the Postmenopause." *Update*, p. 789.

1981: "Premenstrual Syndrome." *British Journal of Psychiatry*, p. 199.

17 April 1982: "Legal implications of premenstrual syndrome." *World Medicine*.

November 1982: "Postnatal Depression." Letter in *British Medical Journal*.

1982: "Overview of premenstrual syndrome." Chapter in *Behavior and the Menstrual Cycle*. R. Friedman, Ed. Marcel Dekker, New York.

1982: "Premenstrual syndrome and its treatment." *International Medicine*, vol. 2, no. 2, pp. 10–13.

1982: "What is this PMS?" *Journal of the Royal College of General Practice*, pp. 717–719.

1983: "Premenstrual syndrome: a new criminal defense?" *California Western Law Review*, vol. 18, no. 2, pp. 268–286. Joint authorship with Lawrence Taylor.

1983: "Migraine." Reference Book Royal College of General Practitioners, pp. 315–316.

1984: "The depression of PMS and menstrual distress." *Mimms*, March 1984, pp. 32–33.

1984: "Menstruation and migraine." *Migraine Matters*, vol. 2, no. 1, pp. 6–8.

1984: "Diagnosis and clinical features of premenstrual syndrome." Chapter in *Premenstrual Syndrome and Dysmenorrhoea*. M. Y. Dawood, Ed. Urban, and Schwarzburg.

18 May 1985: "Pyridoxine overdose in premenstrual syndrome." *The Lancet*, p. 1168.

June 1985: "Progesterone prophylaxis used successfully in postnatal depression." *The Practitioner*, vol. 229, p. 507.

September 1985: "Erythema multiforme associated with menstruation." *Journal of the Royal Society of Medicine*, vol. 78, p. 787.

1985: "Menstrual stress." *Stress Medicine*, vol. 1, pp. 127–133.

1985: "Natural Progesterone and Antihypertensive Action." *British Medical Journal*, vol. 200, p. 1078.

March 1986: "Vitamins: a new perspective." *Mimms Magazine*.

1986: "Premenstrual syndrome." *Hamline Law Review*, vol. 9, no. 1, pp. 143–154.

1986: "Should premenstrual syndrome be a legal defence?" Chapter in *Premenstrual Syndrome: Ethical Implications in a Bio-Behavioural Prospective*. B. F. Carter and B. E. Ginsburg, Eds.

January 1987: "Nasal absorption of progesterone in women." *British Journal of Obstetrics and Gynaecology*, vol. 94, pp. 84–88. Joint authorship with M. E. Dalton, D. R. Bromham, C. L. Ambrose, and J. Osborne.

1987: "The efficacy of progesterone suppositories as a contraception in women with severe PMS." *British Journal of Family Planning*, vol. 13, pp. 87–89. Joint authorship with M. E. Dalton and K. Guthrie.

1987: "Premenstrual syndrome and thyroid." Accepted for publication by *Integrative Psychiatry*.

1987: "Characteristics of pyridoxine overdose neuropathy syndrome." *Acta Neurologica Scandinavia*, vol. 76, pp. 8–11. Joint authorship with M. J. T. Dalton. Awarded Cullen Prize.

1987: "What is this PMS?" Chapter in *The Psychology of Women—Ongoing Debates*. Mary Roth Walsh, Ed. Yale University Press.

1987: "Incidence of PMS in twins." *British Medical Journal*, vol. 295, pp. 1027–8. Joint authorship with M. E. Dalton and K. Guthrie.

June 1987: "Trial of progesterone vaginal suppositories in the treatment of premenstrual syndrome." Letter in *American Journal of Obstetrics and Gynecology*, vol. 156, no. 6, p. 1555.

1987 Commentary on: "Premenstrual syndrome and thyroid dysfunction." *Integrative Psychiatry*, vol. 5, pp. 179–193.

September 1988: "Women's Problems in General Practice." *Stress Medicine*, vol. 4, no. 3, p. 183.

1988: "Treating the premenstrual syndrome." *British Medical Journal*, vol. 297, p. 490.

1988: "Progesterone for premenstrual exacerbations of asthma." *The Lancet*, 2; 8912 p. 684.

1988: "Premenstrual Syndrome." *Health Visitor, vol.* 61, 7, no. p. 199.

September 1989: "Successful prophylactic progesterone for idiopathic postnatal depression." *International Journal of Prenatal & Perinatal Studies.*

October 1989: "PMS: Critique of a Study." *Medical Monitor.* pp. 33–34.

1989: "Postpartum depression & bonding." *International Journal of Prenatal & Perinatal Studies*, pp. 225–226.

May 1990: "Hypothesis: the aetiology of premenstrual syndrome is with the progesterone receptors." *Medical Hypothesis.*

1990: "Do progesterone receptors have a role in PMS?" *International Journal of Prenatal & Perinatal Studies.*

1990: "Premenstrual Syndrome and Postnatal Depression." *Health and Hygiene*, vol. 11, p. 199–201.

March 1991: "Birth of the Blues: Postnatal Depression." *Chemist & Druggist*, pp. 34–36.

1991: "Premenstrual Syndrome: An Alternative View." *British Journal of Hospital Medicine*, vol. 45.

1991: "DMPA and Bone Density." Letter co-authored with M. J. T. Dalton, *British Medical Journal*, vol. 303, p. 855.

1992: "Diet of Women with Severe Premenstrual Syndrome and the Effect of Changing to a Three-Hourly Starch Diet." with W. Holton. *Stress Medicine*, vol. 8, pp. 61–65.

1992: "Early Detection of Pre-eclampsia." *American Journal of Obstetrics and Gynecology*, vol. 167, no. 5, pp. 1479–1480.

1993: "Epidemiology of Premenstrual Symptoms." Letter in *Journal of Clinical Epidemiology*, vol. 46, no. 4, pp. 406–407.

1994: "Progesterone and Glucose Metabolism." with W. M. Holton. *British Journal of Family Planning*, vol. 19, suppl. pp. 4–5.

1994: "Postnatal Depression and Prophylactic Progesterone." *British Journal of Family Planning*, vol. 19, suppl. pp. 10–12.

1994: "Progesterone as a Contraceptive in Severe PMS Sufferers," with M. Steward. *British Journal of Family Planning*, vol. 19, suppl. pp. 23–24.

1994: "Effect of Oral Administration of Corticosterone on Neonatal and Juvenile Rat Physical and Locomotor Development," with G. Pavlovska-Teglia, G. Stodulski, L. Svendson, and J. Hau.

1998: "Alternatives to Hormone Replacement Therapy." *British Journal of Therapy and Rehabilitation*, June, vol. 3.

1998: "Premenstrual Syndrome." Chapter in *Encyclopaedia of Mental Health* (California, Academic Press).

1998: "Psychological Implications of the Menopause." *British Journal of Therapy and Rehabilitation*, June, vol. 3.

APPENDIX

—— ❧ ——

PMS Clinics and Support Groups in the U.S.

This appendix is compiled from information received up to January 1999, but may not be comprehensive. The first list comprises clinics with a medical director who accepts that PMS is a hormonal disease. The second list includes the names of clinics, self-help groups, and other organizations with a nonmedical director whose approach to PMS may be psychological, nutritional, educational, or herbal. Some are lay organizations that act as local referral agencies, others organize self-help groups, and most are able to put PMS sufferers in touch with physicians who understand progesterone therapy. Both lists are organized alphabetically by state and by zip code within each state.

Those marked with a † have a member of the staff who has attended at least one lecture by Dr. Dalton. Those marked with an * have a member of the staff who has attended a 2–4 day training course with Dr. Dalton.

While every attempt has been made to make these lists useful, they cannot remain comprehensive or up-to-date.

These addresses and related information are only supplied as a service to the reader seeking further information. The inclusion of any group does *not* constitute a recommendation or endorsement of any kind by the author or the publisher. The author and publisher cannot be held liable for any results from self-treatment or treatment at any of the facilities listed in this book.

GROUPS WITH A MEDICAL DIRECTOR

Alaska

†The Health Care Center   (907) 562-7643
5001 Arctic Blvd., Ste. 100   fax: (907) 561-1893
Anchorage AK 99503   W. Scott Kiester, D.O.
Jan Kiester, R.N.

Arizona

*Gynecology Ltd.   (602) 264-3267
3330 N. 2nd Street, Ste. 211   fax: (602) 264-0660
Phoenix AZ 85012   Donald E. Lee, M.D.

Mountain View Pharmacy   Evelyn Timmons
10565 North Patum Boulevard   (800) 602-942-7065
Paradise Valley AZ 85253   (800) 602-948-9489

California

†PMS Center   (310) 276-1151
9201 Sunset Blvd., Ste. 708   fax: (310) 276-5782
Los Angeles CA 90069   Lloyd Byron Craig, M.D.

Connie Chein, M.D.   (310) 274-8310
9242 Olympic Blvd.   fax: (310) 274-7025
Beverly Hills CA 90212

Saint Mark Medical Group   (213) 587-1175
7648 Seville Avenue   (213) 587-7358
Huntington Park CA 90255   Amal Y. Zaky, M.D.
Emad M. Gharghoury

* PMS Treatment Clinic   (626) 447-0679
150 N. Santa Anita, Ste. 755   fax: (626) 447-8749
Arcadia CA 91006   Holly Anderson, Director
Linda Crawford, D.O.

* PMS Medical Clinic of   (626) 798-9431
  So. Cal.   fax: (626) 798-0156
2595 E. Washington Blvd.,   Thomas L. Riley, M.D.
  Ste. 106   Rayne Dawson, PAC
Pasadena CA 91107

San Diego PMS Clinic   (619) 297-3311
591 Camino de la Reina,   Lori A. Futterman,
  Ste. 533   R.N., Ph.D.
San Diego CA 92108   M. E. Ted Quigley, M.D.

*PMS of Orange County   (949) 496-7255
32545-B Golden Lantern Rd.,   fax: (949) 443-1407
  Ste. 252   Frank William Varese, M.D.
Dana Point CA 92629

*June A. Engle, M.D., M.S.   (925) 866-9529
5201 N. Canyon Road, Ste. 320   fax: (925) 866-8947
San Ramon CA 94583

Humboldt County Health   (707) 445-6200
  Department   (707) 268-2110
Women's Health Services Gena C. Pennington, M.D.
529 I Street
Eureka CA 95501

Northcountry Clinic   (707) 822-2481
785 18th Street   fax: (707) 822-3656
Arcata CA 95521   Lynn Szabo, PA-C

Florida
The Florida PMS Clinics Inc.   (305) 687-6500
15490 NW 7th Ave., Ste. 207   Vera Selmore, M.D.
Miami FL 33169

Public Health Center for Women   (904) 354-3614
515 West 6th Street
Jacksonville FL 32206

Women's Resource Center
1717 North East Street
Pensacola FL 32501

(850) 434-4054

Georgia
Bernard Mlaver Medical Clinic
4480 N. Shallowford Road, #222
Atlanta GA 30338

(770) 395-1600
fax: (770) 395-9047
Bernard Mlaver, M.D.

Illinois
*Center for Women's Health
1900 West Ogden Ave.
Aurora IL 60505

(630) 978-6290
(708) 844-3412
William H. Woodruff,
M.D., Ob-Gyn
Peg Sechrest, RNC

Iowa
Women's Health Center
1010 Fourth Street SW
Mason City IA 50401

(515) 422-6000
fax: (515) 422-6007
Susan Sieh, M.D.
Maxine Brinkman, R.N.
Nancy Lindgren, MSW

Michigan
†William Beaumont Hospital
Department of Ob/Gyn
3601 W. 13 Mile Road
Royal Oak MI 48073

(248) 551-5000
fax: (248) 551-3616
William Keye, M.D.

Premenstrual Institute

(248) 424-9255 /
(248) 424-9030
Michael L. Berke, M.D., P.C.
Abraham Blumer, M.D., P.C.
Ronald G. Zack, M.D., P.C.

Missouri
*PMS Program Center
939 Gardenview Office Parkway
St. Louis MO 63141

(314) 997-3333
Joseph G. Nouhan, M.D.
Patricia C. Coughlin, Ph.D.
Catherine L. Fox

Joe A. Gardner, M.D., Inc.   (417) 782-2660
3302 Macintosh Circle, Ste. 303   Joe A. Gardner, M.D.
Joplin MO 64804

Montana
Planned Parenthood of Billings   (406) 248-3636
721 N. 29th Street   fax: (406) 245-8182
Billings MT 59101   Clayton McCracken, M.D.

New York
The Premenstrual Symptoms Program   (212) 241-0163
Mount Sinai Medical Center   fax: (212) 369-6817
P.O. Box 1228   email: sk2@academic.mssm.edu
One Gustave L. Levy Place   Stephanie Klein Stern,
New York NY 10128   M.D., Director

The National Council on   (212) 746-6967
   Women's Health (NCWH)   fax: (212) 746-8691
1300 York Avenue, Box 52   Sally Faith Dorfman, M.D.,
New York NY 10021   MSHSA, Medical Advisor
                                            for the Gynecologic
                                               Health Center

North Carolina
PMS Clinic   Marchia Szewczyk, M.D.
Dept. of Family & Community
   Medicine
Bowman Gray School of
   Medicine
300 S. Hawthorne Road
Winston-Salem NC 27130

Ohio
*PMS and Menopausal   (419) 422-6717
   Treatment Center   Mahendra C. Parekh, M.D.,
300 W. Wallace, Ste. B-4   FACOG
Findlay OH 45840

Oregon
PMS Treatment Center
10373 NE Hancock
P.O. Box 20998
Portland OR 97220-0998

(503) 251-4224
Phil Alberts, M.D., FACOG
Suzanne L. Alberts, RNC
Michael S. Alberts, Ph.D., M.D.

Pennsylvania
Christiane M. F. Siewers, M.D.
135 Freeport Road
Pittsburgh PA 15215

(412) 782-2992
fax: (412) 782-3108
Pat Park
Christiane M. F. Siewers, M.D.

University of Pennsylvania
Department of Ob/Gyn
U of Pennsylvania Hospital
3400 Spruce Street
Philadelphia PA 19104

(215) 662-3230
fax: (215) 349-5893
Ellen W. Freeman, Ph.D.
Steven J. Sondheimer, M.D.

Tennessee
*Vanderbilt University PMS Program
Center for Fertility &
   Reproductive Research
Vanderbilt U. Medical Center North
Nashville TN 37232

(615) 322-6957
Joel T. Hargrove, M.D.

Utah
Deborah F. Robinson, M.D.
324 10th Avenue, Ste. 154
Salt Lake City UT 84103

(801) 321-5151
fax: (801) 321-3598

PMS Specialists of Utah
501 Chipeta Way, Ste. 1250
Salt Lake City UT 84108

(801) 584-2038
fax: (801) 582-8471
Richard Shanteau, M.D.
Leanne Geigle

Wisconsin
Heinz Psychological Services
PMS Program
2103 Heights Drive
Eau Claire WI 54701

(715) 834-3171
fax: (715) 834-3174
Sharon A. Heinz, MSE

GROUPS WITH NO MEDICAL DIRECTOR

California

*Parenting Center	(310) 476-8561
Stephen S. Wise Temple	fax: (310) 472-9395
15500 Stephen S. Wise Drive	Marilyn Brown
Los Angeles CA 90077	Kathryn Nessel

Illinois

*PMS Holistic Center of Illinois	(708) 520-3822
942 Twisted Oak Lane	Linaya Hahn
Buffalo Grove IL 60089	

Minnesota

*PMS Discovery, Support,	(612) 472-5311
Center and Training	Joy Bennet, M.A., Director
5023 Edgewater Drive	
Mound MN 55364	

PMS, Postpartum Depression,	(612) 922-5767
and Menopause Clinic	Jane A. Trimble, M.S.,
7101 York Avenue South	R.N., C.S.
Minneapolis MN 55435	

Montana

Blue Mountain Clinic	(406) 721-1646
1610 North California	fax: (406) 543-9890
Missoula MT 59802	Sally Mullen, Director
	Louise Flanagan, R.N.

Oklahoma

University of Oklahoma	(405) 271-8717
College of Medicine	fax: (405) 271-8547
Dept. of Ob/Gyn	Norma Leslie, Ph.D., ARNP
P.O. Box 26901,	
4SP Room 503	
Oklahoma City OK 73190	

Oregon
Robert Sklovsky, Naturopathic
   Physician
6910 SE Lake Road
Milwaukee OR 97267

(503) 654-3938
fax: (503) 654-5829
Robert Sklovsky,
Pharm. D., N.D., P.C.

Texas
Ray's Pharmacy, Inc.
400 S. Main
Mansfield TX 76063

(800) 255-7135
fax: (817) 473-6749
Danny Ray, R.Ph.
Gary Wynn, R.Ph.

Prof. Compounding Centers
   of America
10925 Kinghurst, Ste. 520
Houston TX 77099

(800) 331-2498
fax: (800) 874-5760
David Sparks, R.Ph.
Lawson Kloesel, R.Ph.
Andrew Glasnapp, R.Ph.

Wisconsin
Metabolic Analysis Labs, Inc.
1202 Ann Street
Madison WI 53713

(608) 255-2491
fax: (608) 257-3015
A. L. Shug, Ph.D.
K. J. Shug

*PMS Access
(Madison Pharmacy
   Associates)
P.O. Box 9326
429 Gammon Place
Madison WI 53715

(800) 222-4PMS
(National Women's Hotline)
fax: (608) 833-7412
Marla Ahlgrimm, R.Ph.
David Myers, R.Ph.
Debra Short

*Women's International Pharmacy
5708 Monona Drive
P.O. Box 6468
Madison WI 53716-0468

Wallace L. Simons, R.Ph.

National PMS Hotline
(800) 344-4PMS (4767)

How To Locate a Compounding Pharmacist

There are compounding pharmacies all over the country and locating one nearby is not difficult. If there is no compounding pharmacy nearby, nearly all transactions can be carried out via mail, phone and/or fax.

The easiest way to locate a compounding pharmacist is to contact the International Academy of Compounding Pharmacists (IACP) or the Professional Compounding Centers of America, Inc. (PCCA).

PCCA provides compounding pharmacists with support in the form of training, equipment, chemicals, and technical consultation on difficult compounding problems. At present, more than 2400 compounding pharmacists in the U.S., Canada, Australia, and New Zealand are members of PCCA. For more information about PCCA, including a list of compounding pharmacists:

Telephone: (800) 331-2498   fax: (800) 874-5760
Internet: www.thecompounders.com

Contact the IACP at:
PO Box 1365   (800) 927-4227
Sugar Land TX 77487   fax: (281) 495-0602

Index

295